Eating for Beauty

FOR WOMEN AND MEN

*Introducing a Whole New Concept of Beauty
What It Is, and How You Can Achieve It*

Eating for Beauty...

A system for acheieving radiant, glowing skin and lustrious hair.
A complete youth-enhancing diet and superfood program

DAVID WOLFE

WWW.DAVIDWOLFE.COM

"Beauty will save the world."

— *Fyodor Dostoyevsky*

Printed on recycled paper by
Sunfood Publishing (www.sunfood.com)
P.O. Box 900202
San Diego, CA 92190 U.S.A.

Call or write for more information:
1-888-729-3663

Eating For Beauty is distributed by North Atlantic Books. (www.northatlanticbooks.com)

First Edition: March 30, 2002
Second Edition: August 6, 2003
Third Edition: August 6, 2007

ISBN-13: 978-1-55643-732-8
ISBN-10: 1-55643-732-3

A Note To The Reader

Each lesson in this book contains facts, concepts, and ideas that build upon the lesson before it. Therefore, on the first time through, we urge the reader to avoid skipping the lessons. The reading will surely prove most fruitful if you begin at the Table of Contents and read straight through.

All poems are the author's work.

Many of the products mentioned in this book are available from Sunfood Nutrition (www.sunfood.com). Sunfood Nutrition (www.sunfood.com) is committed to providing the most incredible and unique health and beauty foods and products available in the world today. All products are inspired by principles of sustainable organic agriculture, heart-centered ethics and morality, and living in harmony with nature. All products are diligently researched and tested before they are chosen for distribution.

Disclaimer

This book is sold for information purposes only. Neither the author nor the publisher will be held accountable for the use or misuse of the information contained in this book. This book is not intended as medical advice. The author and publisher of this work are not medical doctors and do not recommend the use of mineral-deficient foods, drugs, or medicines to achieve beauty and to alleviate health challenges. Because there is always some risk involved, the author, publisher, and/or distributors of this book are not responsible for any adverse effects or consequences of any kind resulting from the use or misuse of any suggestions or procedures described hereafter.

Outside Cover Art:
Ken Seaney, Amy Gayheart

Kirlian Photography:
Christopher Wodtke (www.kirlian.com)

Cover Photo: The Cover Photo of *Eating For Beauty* is of Rainbeau Mars. Rainbeau is an actress, teacher, yogini, and mother. She is the international ambassador for Adidas' new mind/body apparel line. She has her own series of best-selling yoga DVDs and is also acting in positive film and television projects. Rainbeau has written columns and articles for several yoga and health magazines, and she is currently finishing a book full of holistic beauty secrets. Her days are filled with inspiring herself and those around her to be the best they can be as human beings, mothers, healthy homemakers, and realizers of extraordinary goals. She wants everyone to know that beauty and indulgence can co-exist with generosity and compassion.

www.rainbeaumars.com

Total Book Design and Text Layout:
David Wolfe and Print.Net, Inc.

Acknowledgments

There are dozens of pages of people I could list here to thank. You all know who you are. I would like to name one person, however — my Mom. Thanks Mom for bringing me into this world! I love you!

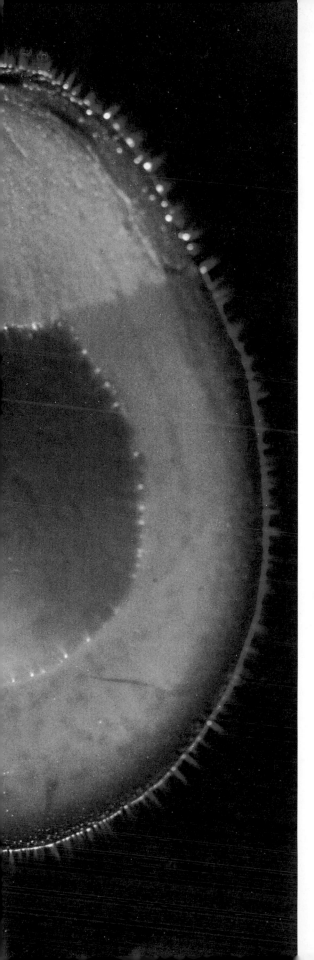

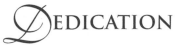

OTHER BOOKS & PROJECTS BY DAVID WOLFE

BOOKS
The Sunfood Diet Success System
Naked Chocolate
Amazing Grace

AUDIO PROGRAMS
Available from www.thebestdayever.com

AVALON CLOTHING LINE
DESIGNED BY DAVID WOLFE AND ANITA ARZE
Eco-Toltec Hemp Pants and Shirts
Eco-Toltec Ponchos

COMPACT DISC MUSIC
This Cooked Planet by The Healing Waters Band
10 original songs
All Is One by The Healing Waters Band
12 original songs
(David Wolfe is the drummer and executive producer)
www.thehealingwatersband.com

VIDEO AND DVD
Exotic Nutrition *(DVD series)* with David Wolfe

David Wolfe is the executive producer of
Raw Yoga with Kim Toledo *(video)*

DAVID WOLFE WEBSITES
www.sunfood.com
www.davidwolfe.com
www.thebestdayever.com
www.ftpf.org

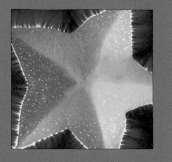

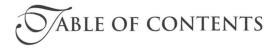

TABLE OF CONTENTS

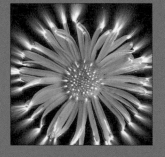

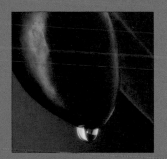

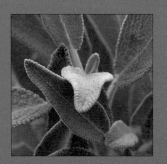

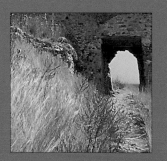

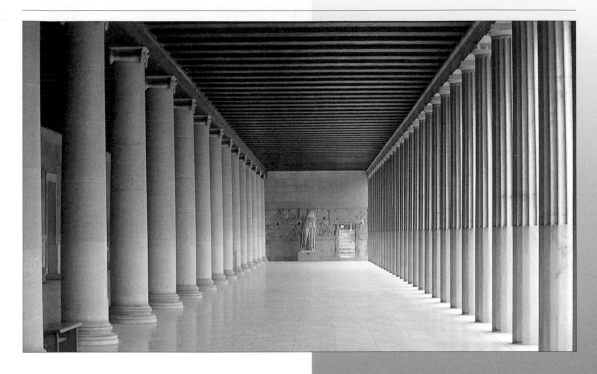

INTRODUCTION

Greetings and Welcome!

*This book
is about how
to become
more beautiful,
not just maintain beauty
or even how to slow
the aging process.*

*This message
is about rejuvenation
at the deepest level.*

*It is about
recreating
one's internal and
external appearance.*

The word "beauty" is derived through French to its Latin root of "bonus," meaning "good." The desire for beauty is not only good and natural, but is in fact one of the most divine attributes; it is one of our sacred possessions. The greatest aspirations in life are to elevate ourselves to the highest state of physical, mental, and spiritual beauty; to discover and draw out our dormant levels of excellence; and to become strongly attractive — magnetic.

The ability to cultivate and appreciate beauty greatly enhances one's ability to heal and enjoy life at every level. The fulfillment derived from the enjoyment and creation of beauty seems to be unmatched by any of life's quests.

As you delve into this book you will discover how to create beauty within yourself through diet and other complementary factors. We will explore the role of yoga, beauty sleep, and the psychology of beauty; yet, primarily, this book is about the way to eat for beauty.

Different foods fuel different types of thoughts; different foods fuel different potentials for success; different foods fuel different destinies or destinations in life — what you are eating now is leading you to a certain destination. Where are you headed with your current diet?

The whole process of digestion is related to our appearance. The manifestation of our genetic and spiritual blueprint is a result of whatever we eat, assimilate, and eliminate.

Not all diets are created equal, as we know. If a certain diet contains the elements of charisma, charm, and magnetism, then it favors beauty building.

One who eats for beauty becomes a work of art in progress. Nature's paint brush immediately sets about applying food-mineral cosmetics to the inner tissues, which become visible externally in the warm, vivid, youthful freshness of the hair, nails, and skin.

One of life's greatest goals is to design a proper diet for ourselves: one that makes us feel incredible in each moment, leads us to limitless beauty, and increases longevity. My desire is to provide you with clues and tools (*not rules*) on how to do this.

People often hear conflicting nutritional advice, roll their eyes, and decide they might as well eat what they want, or what they have always eaten, since the "experts" cannot seem to agree on anything anyway. I know you will find that the information in this book will resonate with your common sense. Always trust your common sense, regardless of what the "experts" say. Judge by results, not by theory.

This book represents my opinions on the beautifying qualities of specific foods based upon experience, science, research, history, intuition, legend, and lore. These foods comprise the core of The Beauty Diet®.

The Beauty Diet® is based on principles of raw nourishment — representing the cutting edge in nutritional science. We now know that raw-plant-foods — especially high-quality fats and oils — can restore elasticity to the tissues. Green-leafy vegetables provide fiber and alkalinity to help keep us clean on the inside. The symmetry of fruit imparts its pattern upon us. Mineralized foods — especially foods high in silicon and magnesium — can restore mineral density to the bones, hair, and teeth.

The Beauty Diet® is simple. You only need to take a few things from this book that you will use. Simple shifts work. The more complicated a diet is, the more likely it is to fail. This is why simple information is provided in this book that you can use immediately.

I have discovered a path toward beauty that can only be described as magical. The food is vibrant, the journey is entertaining. This path toward beauty is what I feel compelled to share with the world.

In providing this information to the world, I aspire to the same type of drive as Michelangelo must have felt when he painted the Sistine Chapel. What an inspiring story! Imagine Michelangelo laying there, on his back, on a precariously high scaffolding, amidst the chill of Italy's winter, the paint dripping into his eyes, doing this at the age of eighty-eight because he had beauty in his soul yet to be shared with the world.

Have you ever been fascinated with a certain subject? I am fascinated by the study of beauty and by the desire to create more beauty in the world. It is sheer fascination with this subject of diet and beauty that has driven me forward to this point through countless exotic adventures, hundreds of health seminars, chance encounters with unique individuals, all-night writing episodes, computer crashes, endless experiments, engaging research, and so much more.

We live in an era where people have realized that artificial diets and chemical treatments for the skin, hair, and body are not as effective as natural methods. The resurgence in the popularity of coconut oil as a moisturizer attests to this. My experience has clearly demonstrated to me that the phenomenal moisturizing properties of organic, cold-pressed coconut oil on the skin cannot be matched by any complicated chemical moisturizer. This is just one example. Natural organic foods and treatments are back — and their popularity is growing at a startling pace.

This book will enlighten and educate you on this trend in beautifying natural foods and treatments. The information within these pages will place the forces of nature squarely in your favor. Nature is always on the side of beauty.

Please remember and take note of the themes alluded to throughout this book. The major theme is that physical beauty is a function of inner cleanliness; it is a function of having healthy skin, hair, nails, and internal connective tissue grown from ideal raw-foods containing high concentrations of the minerals sulfur, silicon, zinc, iron, and manganese. Maintaining the proper acid/alkaline pH balance in the body is a major element of this book. Another theme involves becoming parasite-free by eating foods and herbs that flush out these organisms. Raw antioxidant compounds and foods (*especially those containing vitamins A, C, and E*) that help delay or slow free radical damage to cells and tissues (*thus creating lasting youth*) are thematically referenced. Natural anti-inflammatory foods and food compounds that prevent or reverse facial puffiness are also thematically mentioned throughout these pages.

My desire is to make the human race more beautiful, to bring each person into a more perfect alignment with her/his natural inner self. To further that end I write and publish books like this one, host rejuvenation retreats and conduct seminars all over the world. I hope to see you at a seminar or a retreat sometime soon.

This book is designed for you as an entertaining, educational resource. What amazing gifts we find in books! Books bring so much wonder back into the world. I know this book can inspire you to live more richly, more intensely, more harmoniously and open you to new and more astounding sources of inspiration. *Eating for Beauty* is its own reward, in the moment, and for all one's days.

Enjoy!

David Wolfe
May 2007

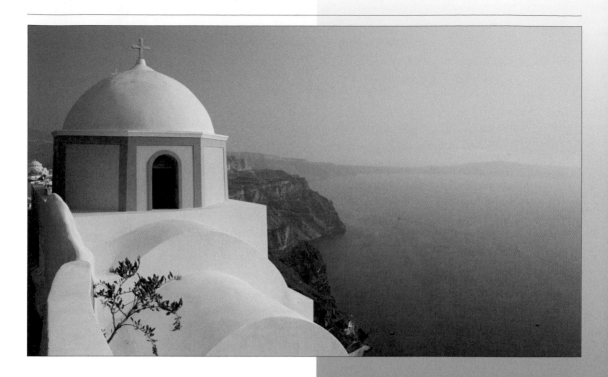

For me, of all eras and cultures, the classical Greek conception of beauty seems to resonate more powerfully than any other. The Greek ideal of beauty has certainly passed — and even surpassed — the test of time.

The ancient Greeks truly tapped into a magical concept. We see, even as far back as Homer's *Iliad*, that beauty was the motivating theme. For these classical Greeks, the hero was always considered beautiful.

The Greek beauty ideal created one of the most fascinating cultures to ever exist on Earth. It gave direction to one of the most extraordinary peoples in history. The classical Greek ideal produced a people of startling appearance. The Roman, Admantius, in his treatise *Physiognomika*, said of the ancient Greeks, "They had square faces, fine lips, straight noses, and powerful eyes with a powerful glittering gaze. They were a people with the most beautiful eyes in the world."

In ancient Greece, a truly beautiful person may have even been honored as a deity after her/his death. Even the half-Greek peoples,

LESSON 1:
COSMIC BEAUTY

Question:
"What do you mean by beauty?"

Answer:
"Perfection of rhythm, balanced perfection of rhythm.

Everything in Nature is expressed by rhythmic waves of light.

Every thought and action is a light-wave of thought and action."

*Walter Russell,
Artist, Architect, Author, Philosopher*

the Egestans, erected a monument to the man held to be the most beautiful Greek in the struggle against the Carthaginians. Sometimes the Greeks would spare an enemy if he impressed them with his beauty. Beauty seemed to them to be a share of divinity — of godliness.

The Roman, Plutarch, left us a telling tale of the Greek reverence for beauty. He described that the Persian general, Masistios, who was killed by the Greeks, was — after his physical beauty had been observed — carried around by the Greek soldiers for general admiration.

In another instance, the Greeks explained that it was the Persian Emperor Xerxes' beauty that justified him on all counts as the true leader of the Persian people.

The Greek conception of beauty continued long after the decline of the city-state *(polis)*. So strong was this ideal, that even when a disintegrated Greece faced the conquering Roman general, T. Quintius Flaminus, whose appearance evoked a memory of its own former greatness, they celebrated him as a national hero due to his dignity and beauty. In Athens, he was treated as one of their own great men.

Symmetry

In his work, the ancient Greek philosopher Plato describes beauty as consisting of proportion and symmetry. Plato understood that the entire human organism is woven together with a mathematical geometrical precision calculated to exact fractions to create a perfect harmony and design.

The late Dr. Herbert Shelton, one of history's most prolific writers on health, a raw-plant-based diet and fasting, was absolutely fascinated with and inspired by the Greek beauty ideal. Dr. Shelton had a memorable definition of beauty. He wrote, "Beauty, in its highest sense, signifies that harmony of proportions, fairness of aspect, and geniality of influence belonging to form, combination, principle, or condition which renders it attractive and pleasing."

Dr. Shelton also wrote, "Beauty, I am fully convinced, is a reflection of excellence, revealing excellence of structure and balance of function; whereas, those defects, disproportions, disharmonies, and asymmetries which make up the various forms of ugliness, signify structural defects and functional imbalances....This, it seems to me, is a fundamental truth of far-reaching importance."

Years ago I saw a Home Box Office *(HBO)* television program in which scientists conducted several experiments trying to qualify beauty. The results led researchers to conclude that beauty is most closely correlated to the phenomenon of symmetry. For example, the more symmetrical an individual's face, the more likely beauty was to be recognized by others in that person.

The conclusion, then, is that symmetry is the first element of beauty. The more exact the symmetry, the more likely it is that beauty will be recognized.

There is no doubt that heredity plays a powerful role in shaping our natural symmetry. People with strong genetic traits of beauty are uniquely blessed. However, even those who have less than excellent genetic gifts will find solace and wonder in the fact that one's bodily form is a work of sculpture in process and no matter what one's genetic code expresses, the power of diet, mind and exercise can reshape and remake the body.

Symmetrical exercises have a subtle but important balancing effect. The practice of yoga helps create more overall symmetry of muscle, tendons, sinews, and organs. In essence, symmetrical exercises involve activities that use the other side of the body than one normally uses. For example, writing with the left hand *(if one is right-handed)*. I play the drums and sometimes practice with my drumset reversed to balance the other side of my body.

A symmetrical mind exercise involves chewing on both sides of the jaw. An ancient yoga technique describes that if one chews fifty-two times on each side of the jaw, this balances both hemispheres of the brain. This is probably due to the fact that the vagus nerve which runs along the temporal mandibular joint *(jaw joint)*, strongly influences over 30% of each brain hemisphere.

Essentially, symmetrical nutrition involves taking in foods that are geometric and based on the golden ratio *(phi)*, such as raw fruits and vegetables. This imparts a balancing pattern upon us.

Electromagnetism and Kirlian Photography

Every now and then we hear of or see someone with a magnetic personality. Even being in the company of such an individual tends to uplift the spirits. This person seems to be surrounded by a refreshing youthful glow. This glow is electromagnetic radiation, the exact same as is visible in Kirlian photography. Harmonious electromagnetic radiation creates an attractive force. This leads us to discover that electromagnetism and beauty are closely aligned.

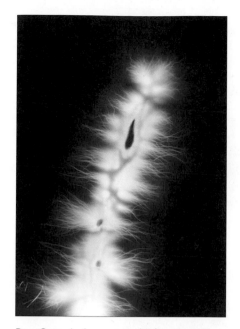

Raw Organic Asparagus *(Kirlian Image)*

We only need to watch a baby to see that we are instinctively attracted to colorful, electromagnetic foods — foods with an aura of vibrant energy.

Kirlian photographs capture the electromagnetic radiation patterns emitted by objects across a wide spectrum of electromagnetic energy. These light patterns are beyond what is visible to the naked eye.

Consider the symmetry and beauty of these Kirlian photographs:

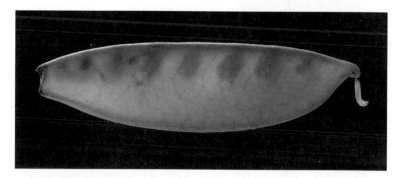

Raw Organic Peapod

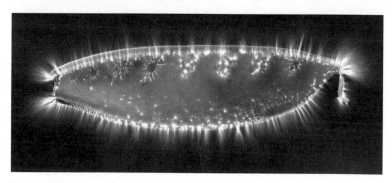

Raw Organic Peapod *(Kirlian Image)*

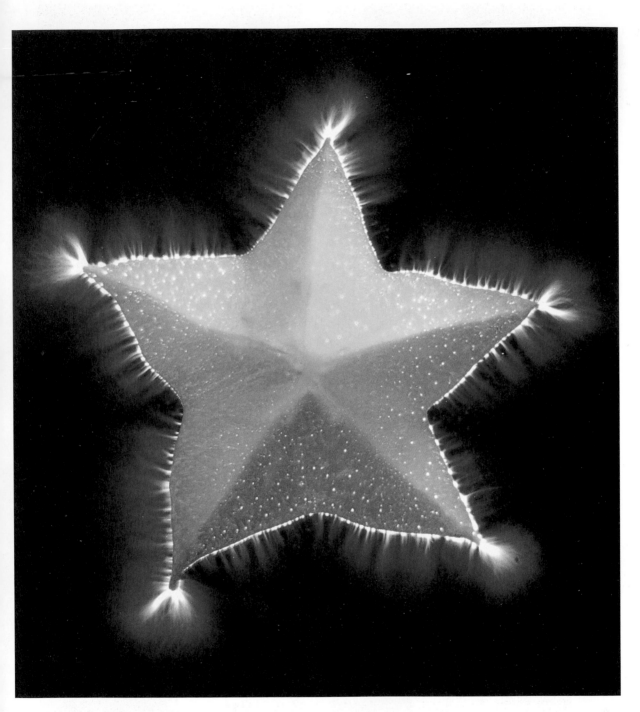

Organic Starfruit *(Kirlian Image)*

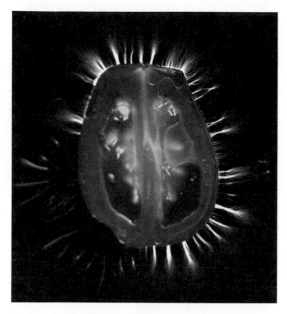

Slightly Cooked Organic Tomato *(Kirlian Image)*

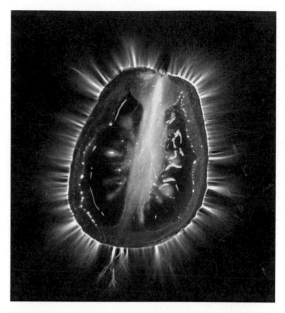

Raw Organic Tomato *(Kirlian Image)*

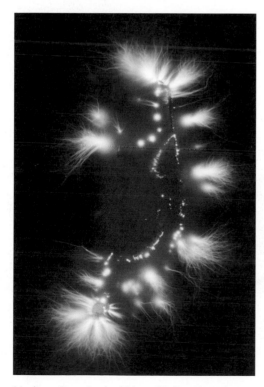

Medium-Rare Cooked Meat *(Kirlian Image)*

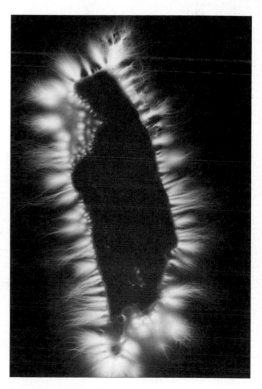

Raw Meat *(Kirlian Image)*

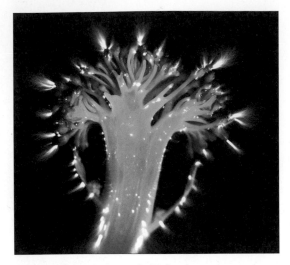

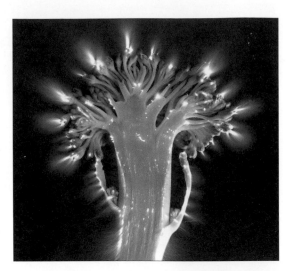

Steamed Organic Broccoli *(Kirlian Image)*

Raw Organic Broccoli *(Kirlian Image)*

From these pictures we can see the intense, vibrant, electromagnetic, and luminescent patterns found in raw-foods as opposed to other foods. When we focus on the elements of beauty and symmetry, we begin to understand that the genre of "raw-plant-food" is the ideal place to start as we begin to design The Beauty Diet®.

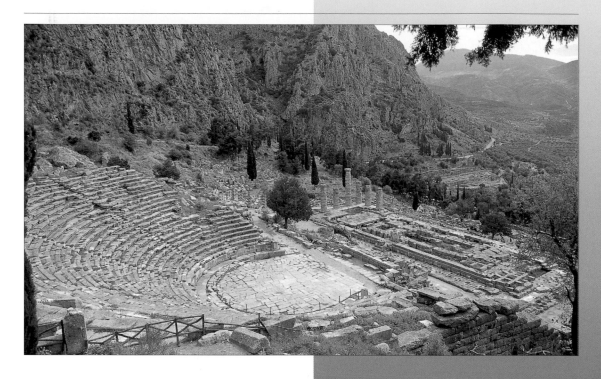

"To attract attractive people, you must be attractive."

*Jim Rohn,
America's Foremost
Business Philosopher*

*B*eauty is such a precious commodity. The potential of beauty is so great that it is never given away freely. "Something for nothing" is against the flow of nature. "Anything worth having is worth working for," was Andrew Carnegie's important insight. If you desire vibrant beauty, you must earn it, step-by-step.

Essentially, beauty is an achievement. To attain it, there are certain things you must do.

Many people are out in the world trying to "get" beautiful. One cannot go out and get beautiful, because beauty is not something you get! Beauty is something you earn by refining the type of person you are becoming. The beautification process is about becoming the type of person who can be beautiful. If you want to become beautiful you have to become that type of person on the inside first and then attract beauty to you. It seems to work this way in all facets of life.

Creating an attractive state of physiology, mental and emotional poise, and spiritual presence *(i.e. becoming a beautiful person)* results from consistent actions. Our physical beauty and attractiveness are directly related to our actions *(habits of behavior)*. The primary behavior we all collectively participate in is the eating of food. The most reliable and consistent action we can apply to achieve beauty is to eat for beauty. What we eat guides us on our path. Eating determines what level of grace and elegance our body will experience moment to moment.

The Power of a Decision

If we can maintain excellent eating habits, then we have truly achieved something extraordinary. Consistency is the key. Our actions are made consistent, not by strict discipline, but rather, they are made so by a refinement of character. The refinement of character begins when one makes a definite decision to target one's life toward a specific destination. So we find, at the root of it all, that lasting beauty, elegance, and charm are attracted by a decision — a decision to eat beautifying food.

We begin by adding. Adding this fruit and that vegetable, this sprout and that seed. The Beauty Diet® is about adding foods into your life. Denial and strict discipline are not part of the program and, for the most part, do not work in the long term. Bringing in nutrient-rich raw-foods and allowing the body to shift automatically at its own pace, so that cooked foods begin to lose their appeal and taste *(when compared to the superior taste of the beauty foods),* is part of the program.

Food Shapes Our Bodies

Just as the crashing waves caress the beach cliffs every day, every night, relentlessly, and thus shape those cliffs ever so subtly, so too do the foods we eat shape our forms subtly, slowly and methodically over time.

Some people have believed that food does not affect them. Picture now that eating is about taking an object that is foreign to our bodies, and putting that inside ourselves. Food is not just a factor that affects us, it is the primary thing that affects us. If what we put inside our bodies does not affect us, what could? Once we know this, then it becomes easier to select foods that add to our strength, spirituality, and beauty, because each meal becomes part of who we are at the deepest level.

Food is exacting. The face is truly a canvas upon which our food choices paint an accurate picture. The body is truly a sculpture, chiseled and polished by our food choices.

"You are what you eat" is such a profound saying that literally everyone knows it. "You are what you eat" is a concept that has been known in every culture and civilization throughout history. It is written into the fabric of the universe. It is a cosmic law. It is a simple law of nature that one may remember each day, and at each meal.

The logic of "You are what you eat" implies that those who wish to become healthier should eat the healthiest foods. Those who wish to beautify themselves should eat the most beautifying foods.

Nutrition is the one thing that is everything. Becoming conscious of the importance of nutrition allows you to begin to chart the direction of change in your life. Becoming conscious of nutrition means that you are becoming aware that little things add up, that consistent actions taken every day begin to take you in a certain direction. Things you do every now and then do not really affect your life — it is what you do consistently, such as eating food, that controls your destiny.

Raw Plant Food

"There is absolutely no nutrient, no protein, no vitamin, no mineral, that we know of, that can't be obtained from plant-based foods."

— *Michael Klaper, M.D., Author, Lecturer*

I found out something in my research. I discovered that just as there are general patterns of nature, of physics, and of chemistry *(quantum physics has discovered that there are no true laws of nature; there are, however, general habit patterns of nature as determined by probabilities),* there are also patterns of success and there are patterns of beauty. There are patterns of phenomenon that are already in place as part of the set-up.

It is important to get clear on nature's set-up. We are all familiar that the world is set up in a certain way — the sun rises, the plants grow, the seasons change. If we throw an apple up, the chances are that it will come down. The universe is governed by general patterns *(even if we do not know what they all are)*. It seems that all human progress and wisdom has been about discovering what those patterns are and coming into an understanding and awareness of those patterns.

The first of these "habits of nature" is called "cause and effect." "Cause and effect" means that each action *(such as eating a meal)* adds up and becomes a cause set in motion leading us to a certain destination. Dietary choices made each day have a cumulative effect; that is why many people have chosen to follow excellent diets. If we are not careful, poor food choices will catch up to us. It is great to remember that, if we start feeling the effects of indigestion, poor digestion, constipation, or lack the feeling of satiation, then we know these "effects" can be remedied by eliminating the "causes." And if we listen to our bodies' messages, we will understand that digestive and other ills are caused by eating the wrong foods. Many people are becoming aware that the world has been set up with certain dietary patterns that have been ideal for us since the moment we first appeared on earth.

During the first ages, humankind subsisted primarily on raw-plant-foods. These included green-leafy foods, as well as nuts, seeds, roots, and fruits, because these were — and still are — the easiest foods to acquire.

Consider the implications of the old story. As the legend goes, it was the forbidden food that caused the fall from grace. We have all had the experience of eating "forbidden foods" *(at late night dinner parties that caused our fall from grace for at least a few days!)*.

People often debate with each other about humans being frugivores, carnivores, omnivores, herbivores, etc. The truth is that human beings will eat anything. Name any plant, animal, worm, insect, or object and odds are that somebody, somewhere has tried to eat it! What becomes fascinating is that when one stops eating "anything," that is the moment when a startling realization occurs — the realization that what we eat deeply and radically affects the way we think, feel, and behave. When one introduces discernment into one's food choices, a physical and spiritual transformation begins to take place.

Someone once said, "I do not know who discovered water, but I can be sure of one thing, it was not a fish." Some things are so obvious, they are so directly in front of us, that they are difficult to see. The value of real, wholesome, raw-plant-based nutrition is one of those things. It has always been here, all around us.

It is nutrient-rich raw-food that places a sparkle in the eye, lustre in the hair, freshness in the skin, and herbal fragrance to the body.

Raw-plant-food is beautiful. Preparing and eating this type of food is an art. Every ingredient is a new color. Each meal is a cloud, a stream, or a flower — a piece of the magnificent painting that you are becoming. Every bite is a detailed brush stroke on your work of art in progress. What we perceive as the world is only a reflection of the work of art we are inside. We find that once we become pure and polished within, everything outside of us also becomes that and more. To me, the raw-food ideal represents not only a way to live in peace, love, and harmony with nature and the animals, but it also represents the highest aspirations of beauty in the human spirit.

Take a moment now to imagine the idealized image of yourself. Get a clear picture of the outstanding potential within you. Could such a god-like ideal be reached by eating junk food? Could such an ideal be reached by anything but the most vibrant, most colorful, most juicy plant foods?

Raw-plant-food contains juice! Juice makes your tissues juicier, juice makes you more juiced about life, and juice allows you to squeeze more juice out of every moment. If you desire beauty, your tissues should have a juicy quality about them.

Realize that the genre of raw-plant-food offers, by far, the largest variety of foods. In reality, 99.99% of all food on Earth, for all creatures, is raw-plant-food. Because this food genre provides the most variety, it also provides the greatest chance of success because we are all biochemically different. One thing is certain, not one specific selection of food works for everyone. Everybody has a different metabolism, and rarely do two people eat the same foods each day. A wonderful benefit of eating raw-plant-foods is the incredible choices that are present; all these choices allow you to access and select any variety of foods that work for you.

Experience has shown that eating raw-foods brings you back into touch with your food instincts, thus allowing you to select more precisely which foods your body needs.

Eating raw-foods increases one's taste sensations and the sensitivity of the taste buds. Many people cannot taste properly for two reasons. The first reason is that their taste buds have been dulled by eating cooked foods. The second reason is that they have a zinc deficiency. Eating zinc-rich raw-foods over time (such as poppy seeds, pumpkin seeds, and pecans) gradually returns one's taste buds back to normal — allowing for more heightened taste pleasures.

A welcome bonus from eating raw-plant-foods is that most meals are ecstatic experiences. And when eating high-quality, fresh, raw-food that the body needs, it feels as if cells in various parts of the body are having orgasms!

What is amazing about the raw-food path is that every step along the way is enjoyable and brings forth its own magic.

The evidence in support of moving toward a raw-plant-based diet is derived from science, natural history, physiology, experience, and common sense. These days, it seems that every health and fitness magazine, television program, and book discusses the benefits of eating vegetables, tomatoes, apples, oranges, berries, raw nuts, raw seeds, sprouts, avocados, wheatgrass juice, etc. These raw-plant-foods are where the magic is found — in the enzyme factor.

Enzymes

The most unique aspect of living, raw-food is its enzyme content. Enzymes begin to be destroyed when food is heated over 120 degrees Fahrenheit.

Enzymes can only be found in living cells, raw-foods, or foods dehydrated at low temperatures. They are particularly beneficial for human health if they come from raw-plant-foods, because plant enzymes provide the most action through various pH (acid/alkaline) conditions in the body.

Enzymes are catalysts. They are transformative elements. They are truly an alchemical symbol of transformation. On a physical level, enzymes help to overcome digestive lethargy. On a spiritual level, enzymes help to overcome life's ruts and setbacks — enzymes overwhelm spiritual stagnation.

If you want things to change for you, if you want to attract and create beauty in your life, you have to do something different than you are doing now. If you desire a different destiny (destination) than relatives and friends who ended up dead broke or dead at the age of 65, then you must do something different now. Food enzymes make the difference.

Enzymes are small proteins. Some nutritionists mistakenly believe that enzymes are destroyed by stomach acid; however, protein cannot be broken down by hydrochloric acid in the stomach. Therefore, enzymes — especially plant enzymes — survive into our intestines and can be absorbed into our tissue system, helping us break down old cooked-food residues and general stagnation.

One of the most enzymatically active locations that exists in nature is found in the mouth of a child eating cooked food. If cooked food is eaten, the body attempts to adapt by increasing the enzyme content of the saliva in order to begin breaking down cooked food as quickly as possible. This adaptation lasts as long as the body has enzyme reserves. As we age, our reserves decrease. Doctor Meyer and his associates at

Michael Reese Hospital, Chicago, found that the enzymes in the saliva of young adults was 30 times stronger than in persons over the age of 69. Without the proper enzymes to break down our foods, we begin to accumulate undigested materials in our system. This leads to weight gain, inflammation, stagnation, digestive distress, and fatigue.

The saliva of a raw-food eater contains far less enzymes than that of a person who eats cooked food. This is because raw-foods contain enzymes, and salivary enzymes are not as necessary for digestion.

Our enzyme reserves correlate to our vitality. Our enzymes and vitality are drained by eating cooked food.

Enzymes found in raw-foods are codes. They tell the food where to go in our bodies. For example, the enzyme erepsin in cucumbers is targeted toward breaking down excessive protein in the kidneys. Therefore, we find that cucumbers are attracted to the kidneys and are excellent for kidney health.

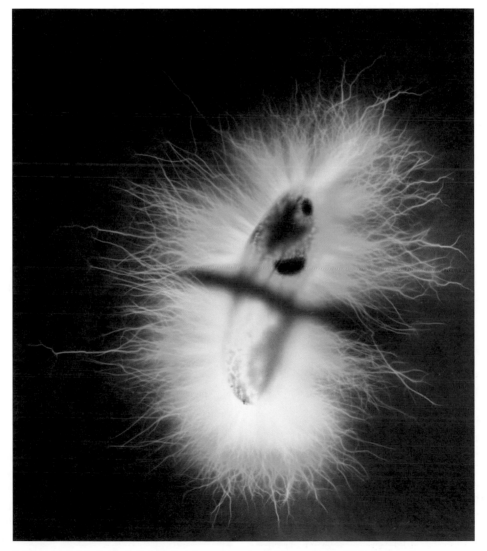

An Enzyme-rich Organic Sunflower Sprout — viewed from above *(Kirlian Image)*

If cooked food is eaten, the body has to re-identify the food, recode it with enzymes, and attempt to deliver it to the proper tissues and organs. This process takes energy and robs vitality. As our vitality decreases, cooked food drains away more and more energy, creating more digestive confusion. As a result, cooked food is often incompletely digested and not properly delivered to the proper tissue site.

Enzymes are not just found in raw-food. They are also found in every cell of your body. Every cell throughout the body has the potential to be a highly-charged battery containing over 4,000 enzymes. Many people have not activated each of these 4,000 enzymes because they do not have enough major and trace minerals in their diet. Minerals, when obtained through their whole raw-food complexes, activate our cellular, metabolic enzyme system. Trace elements *(minerals)* are essential to the proper functioning of enzymes. Minerals give longevity to enzymes. The goal is to increase the minerals and nutrition within each cell so as to activate every enzyme, thus increasing the electromagnetic charge in each cell, causing every cell to resonate in harmony.

At the cellular level, this is truly the picture of perfect health.

— Cooked Food —

"The essential is to get rid of deeply rooted prejudices, which we often repeat without examining them."

— *Albert Einstein*

Have you ever wondered why humans are the only creatures on the Earth who cook their food?

Prometheus — "the contriver" — stole fire from Zeus. The Greek poet Hesiod says that before the time of Prometheus, humankind was exempt from suffering and enjoyed a vigorous youth; and when death did arrive, it was without pain and the eyes were gently closed as in sleep. There is some facet of fire that shifted humanity's state of paradise. I invite you to discover that the shift away from paradise was influenced by cooking. Cooking food, upon close evaluation, appears to contain a core error.

Do you remember your first lesson in junior

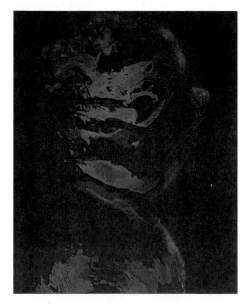

Cooked Cabbage *(Kirlian Image)*

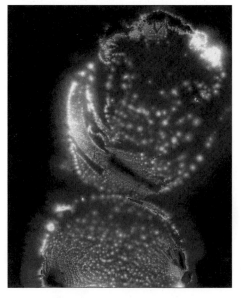

Raw Cabbage *(Kirlian Image)*

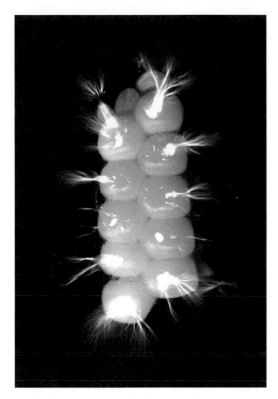

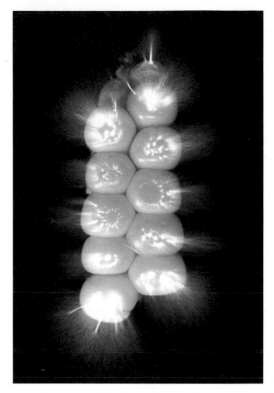

Cooked Organic Corn *(Kirlian Image)*

Raw Organic Corn *(Kirlian Image)*

high school chemistry class? The first thing we did that day was to get out the Bunsen burner and begin heating a test tube. Heat, we learned, causes chemical changes. Cooking causes chemical changes in food. I have heard many naturopathic physicians say that "cooking food creates a host of compounds that the body is not designed to metabolize." Severin Schaeffer, in his book *Instinctive Nutrition*, mentions that cooking a simple potato creates over 400 known, unknown, and potentially dangerous compounds.

Cooking and heating shift the molecular structure of food in both slight and great degrees. These altered molecules may not be the ideal building blocks for our tissues. However, since our bodies are always doing the best they can, they will *(if given nothing else)* incorporate these altered or cooked molecules into our bodily structure.

Eating food that has been heated above a certain temperature *(slightly under 200 degrees Fahrenheit)* causes a pathogenic response in the body called leukocytosis whereby white blood cells *(leukocytes)* are actually used to digest food much as they would attack a foreign substance. This statement has been confirmed in hundreds of experiments and is based on the research of the Swiss scientist Paul Kouchakoff.

It has been said, "one half of human ailments are caused by bad cooking" *(and to this I add the other half are caused by good cooking!)*.

Not all foods are created equal, as we are discovering. Certain types of food add to beauty, while certain other types of food definitely detract from beauty.

When one is eating for beauty, the burdensome, heavily-cooked diet is left behind.

Certainly someone could eat cooked and processed foods and still be beautiful. However, such a person could never become MORE beautiful eating such a diet. The situation is similar with chronic disease. One could survive such a condition for a time on cooked and processed food, but one could be quite challenged trying to reverse the condition on such a diet. The present-day diet is detrimental to increasing beauty, charisma, health, prosperity and youthfulness. Our higher consciousness thrives only in a body filled with youthful, supple, juicy raw-foods containing a high quantity of minerals.

Living Liquids

One of the most important characteristics of a healthy eating plan is to eat foods that the body can readily turn into a liquid.

The juice of the plant, like the blood of the body, contains all the essential elements that build and nourish. The entire premise behind digestion is to take food and convert it into a liquid to be passed through the intestinal villi into the bloodstream. The human body is truly an advanced juicing machine.

Cooked foods contain no vital juices. The first thing that is lost when food is cooked, even before enzymes are lost, is water. Anything that is cooked is devoid of living water. So the body has a challenging time converting cooked food into a usable form to be absorbed. This is because everything we eat must be converted into a liquid for it to nourish us.

Now imagine how much energy it takes to convert bread into a liquid! How much energy is required to turn a steak into a liquid? With this perspective, we clearly see why digestion is the #1 energy drain. There is no other life-process that requires as much energy as digestion.

Thus, we see that the major difference between cooked food and raw-food is that one is a dead solid, and the other is a living liquid. This makes it much easier to see which is easier *(and which is more difficult)* to digest.

Refined Sugar and Cooked Starch

It seems that the most unhealthy-looking people eat refined sugar and white flour products. Candy, sweets, cakes and sodas destroy the teeth and complexion while adding layers of unwanted weight. Starchy cooked carbohydrates make the skin dry and pasty-white in color.

Cooked starchy foods such as bread, rice, pasta, rice cakes, potato chips, corn chips, baked potatoes and sweet soy drinks tend to be low in minerals and high in sugar. This is the exact characteristic we should avoid in food. This characteristic strongly influences blood sugar levels making cooked starchy foods quite addicting.

Types of food containing high carbohydrates *(sugars)* and low amounts of minerals also run minerals out of the body. This is because minerals are heavily used by the pancreas to create enzymes to digest cooked food and to create insulin to balance the blood sugar fluctuations caused by eating starchy food.

This characteristic of a food containing high carbohydrates *(sugar)* and low minerals can lead to a fungus, yeast *(candida)* and mold overgrowth in the body. Because candida is such a common issue, I dedicated an entire section to it in my book *The Sunfood Diet Success System*.

The low quantity of minerals found in cooked starchy carbohydrates is partly due to hybridization of crops and abysmal commercial farming practices. Standard commercial farming occurs in mineral-deficient soil using weak seeds. Without minerals and strong genetics, plants become subject to pestilence *(insects, fungus, mold, etc.)*. This has brought about the destructive use of pesticides in a fruitless attempt to remedy the situation. These foods, even after cooking, processing, and packaging are still subject to attack by fungus, yeast, and mold. When digested, these foods can feed fungus, yeast, and mold already within the digestive system.

Everything that we eat should be as densely mineralized as possible; therefore, we should eat organic foods grown in mineral-rich soils grown from strong seed strains.

Cooked Oil and Fat

My experience has demonstrated to me that cooked oil and fat — especially cooked vegetable oil, margarine, and animal fat — are the most detrimental of all foods. Cooked oil, margarine, and animal fat are particularly destructive because they are not miscible with water. Since we are a water-based lifeform, this makes the metabolization of cooked oil difficult at best. Cooked oil, margarine, and animal fat are inflammatory to the tissues, cloud the brain, harm the cardiovascular system, and accelerate the aging process.

Cooked oily foods (anything from fried chicken to the typical stir fry to potato chips) negatively affect our skin's health and lead to acne and body pimples. Cooked oil, margarine, and fried foods are absolutely detrimental to the complexion.

Cooking and Vitamins

Vitamin A, D, E, and K dissolve in fat (they are fat-soluble), hence these are lost in frying when fats/oils are corrupted.

High temperatures destroy vitamin C and most of the B vitamins, including vitamin B12.

A deficiency of vitamin A seems to be associated with acne and skin disorders. The plant-form of vitamin A (beta-carotene) is found in arugula, watercress, broccoli, spinach, dandelion, cantaloupe, and carrots, along with many other foods.

Vitamin E is completely corrupted by frying. A deficiency of vitamin E is related to indigestion and heart disease. The best plant source of vitamin E is olive oil.

Raw vitamin E (tocopherol) has long been considered a healing factor in reversing heart disease and a topical panacea for wrinkles and facial lines. High-grade vitamin E compounds called tocotrienols are the best supplemental source of vitamin E. Tocotrienols were at one time more than $4,000 a bottle. Now they are down to $50 per bottle. In nature, tocotrienols are found in plants (usually seeds). They are extremely heat sensitive and easily destroyed. They are currently available in an edible powder form. The powder contains alpha-tocotrienols, which are 40 to 50 times more powerful (in repairing skin damage, protecting the heart, and as antioxidants) than regular vitamin E. The powder also contains delta-tocotrienols, which are 200 times more powerful than regular vitamin E.

Rancid Oils

Cooking oil creates highly toxic trans-fatty acids. Trans-fatty acids may be absorbed into the body's cell membranes, causing them to become porous and weak.

Consider all cooked or exposed oils to be rancid. Rancid oils are not detectable by taste, unless there is some protein in the oil. For example, rancid milk is easy to detect, because it contains quite a bit of protein; when the fat turns rancid, it affects the proteins, causing them to change taste and smell. Rancid flax oil, on the other hand, is not detectable by taste or smell.

The fact that rancid oils suppress the immune system has been recognized by many of the world's leading nutritionists (for more details on this, please read Fats That Heal, Fats That Kill by Udo Erasmus and Free Radicals and Food Additives by P. Addis and G. Warner).

The Free Radical Theory

Cooked oil is the largest cause of free radical damage in the human body. Free radical damage has come to be regarded as the primary cause of aging.

The free radical theory was first proposed by Dr. Denham Harman (Ph.D. and M.D.) at the University of Nebraska back in 1956.

What are free radicals? Free radicals are oxygen molecules that have lost an electron and are thus unstable and reactive. Free radicals are produced by other factors besides cooked oil, including pesticides, cigarette smoke, air pollution, excessive sun exposure, and the natural breakdown of tissues. These radical oxygen molecules bounce around cells and tissues stealing electrons from healthy molecules thus causing damage and creating more free radicals in the process.

Collagen, a protein molecule that gives our skin a youthful, supple look, is especially susceptible to free-radical damage. Free-radical damage can lead to the formation of wrinkles; it can also cause scars to linger and heal improperly. Free-radical damage actually creates a chemical change called "cross-linking." Cross-linked collagen is stiff and inflexible.

Certain nutrients called antioxidants prevent and even reverse free radical damage. Antioxidants may be in the form of fatty acids *(raw fats and/or cold-pressed oils)*, minerals *(manganese, selenium)*, vitamins *(A, C, E)*, and complex biological compounds *(pycnogenol, tocotrienols, unheated THC)*. Antioxidants prevent and reverse damage by simply giving free radicals the electrons they need to become stable. In this way, antioxidants reverse skin inflammation *(i.e. sunburn)* and help to heal scar tissue.

Monounsaturated oils *(olive oil)*, and especially polyunsaturated oils *(corn oil, safflower oil, most vegetable oils, flax oil, hemp oil)*, are very open to oxidation from exposure to light and air, as well as to heat. Oxygen, heat, and light turn normal fats into trans-fatty acids *(these cause degenerative conditions of all types)*, create free radicals *(linked to cancer and aging)*, and cause rancidity. This is why oils must be packed in dark containers, sealed airtight, unheated and consumed in a timely manner. Cooking with monounsaturated or polyunsaturated oils obviously adds heat and also accelerates oxidation.

Common polyunsaturated oils, such as flax oil, hempseed oil, corn oil, canola oil, and safflower oil, are extremely time, light and heat sensitive. Olive oil and butter, though more stable, are also time, light, and heat sensitive. This means they go rancid if left too long and if exposed to light and/or excessive heat.

Butter is more naturally saturated than olive oil; therefore it is better for cooking. However, a far better choice than butter is coconut oil.

As we will discover later in this book, the most beautifying and stable oil is coconut oil *(a saturated fat)*. This is the best butter/oil to cook with, because it is entirely stable up to 170 degrees Fahrenheit.

Other oils and fats that are favorable to beauty, if taken raw, are olive oil, olives, hempseed oil, hemp seeds, macadamia nuts, pine nuts, and pecans.

Animal Products

Ovid, the Roman poet, represents Pythagorus giving the following instructions:

"Take not away the life you cannot give;
For all things have an equal right to live.

Kill noxious creatures where 'tis sin to save:
This only just prerogative we have:

But nourish life with vegetable food,
And shun the sacrilegious taste of blood."

— *Metamorphosis* (Book xv, Line 795)

The truth is that the more researchers understand about the nutrients found in fruits, vegetables, herbs, nuts, and seeds, the more impressed they are with the power of those compounds to retard the bodily breakdown that results in cancer and other chronic degenerative illnesses.

But you never hear any good news about meat. Study after study reveals that meat eating leads to more arthritis, asthma, cancer, diabetes, heart disease, liver disease, kidney problems, and osteoporosis.

Animal Fat and Protein

As we become what we eat, we find that heavy meals of cooked animal protein and fat make the tissues dense and coarse.

There has been much controversy about fish fats and oils. Udo Erasmus reports in his book *Fats That Heal, Fats That Kill* that several species of fish actually contain toxic fats and oils. An example is the toxic cetoleic fatty acid, found in herring, capelin, menhaden, anchovetta, and even in cod liver oil!

Factory-farmed animals contain poor quality oils and fats that, especially when cooked, detract from a beautiful complexion. Animal fats, such as commercial beef and pork, contain a high percentage of the long-chain saturated fats palmitin and stearin. Both of these disfavor beauty. Animal fats also contain the pesticides and toxins the animal was exposed to or ate at the factory farm.

Meat *(unless kosher)* contains urine — kosher meats are drained of blood and urine. The human body, on average, can only process approximately 8 grams of uric acid *(the urine waste of animals, found in meat)* per day. Consider that one 450 gram portion of meat contains 16 grams of uric acid *(urine)*.

Long-chain animal fats are implicated in contributing to a wide variety of health problems, from arteriosclerosis and its increased risks of heart attack and stroke to various cancers and obesity.

Vast numbers of people have now changed their beliefs about protein and animal food. Cooked animal muscles *(meats)* are actually poor-quality protein sources. Cooking coagulates proteins, making them less digestible, more coarse, and more inflammatory.

The best and most assimilable sources of protein are spirulina, blue-green algae, chlorella, hemp seeds, bee pollen, goji berries, Incan berries, flax seeds, pumpkin seeds, durian, olives, sprouts *(all types)*, green vegetables *(especially spinach, watercress, arugula, kale, broccoli, brussel sprouts, collard greens, and parsley)*, powdered grasses, and green super-food products, such as *Pure Synergy* or *Sun Is Shining Superfood*.

Participating in the taking of an innocent animal's life — especially if it is not done in a sacred way as the Native Americans did — makes it difficult to create lasting beauty inside and out. Killing and supporting meat eating has a corrosive effect on the inner consciousness.

Upon a deeper investigation of the soft structure of our internal organs, our teeth *(we have duller canines than even the vegetarian primates)*, and a closer look at our own aversions toward killing and spilling blood, how is it that we could have ever eaten meat at all? The answer is related to an interesting phenomenon: There is a provision amongst the animals through which they are enabled to live on foods their organs were not designed to accommodate.

During their long sea voyages, the Nordics discovered that the lambs on board their ships were induced to eat meat and fish, and upon doing so became habituated to it. Upon arriving on land the lambs no longer desired grass. Horses are often fed fish and can be habituated to enjoy it, even though this is an unnatural food for horses. Frugivorous parrots can be taught to eat and relish animal foods.

Obviously, humans can eat large quantity of animal foods, but it has become increasingly clear that by doing so, a marked decrease occurs in the level of one's health, pleasure, and longevity.

With the exception of the Essenes *(a Judeo-Christian group of raw-foodists)*, as far as we know *(at least since the last flood/pole shift)*, no considerable portion of any human population has, over many generations, ever adopted a specific raw-food diet based upon the wisdom and knowledge of human physiology, superior mental performance, and spiritual goals. In fact, the opposite has most often occurred. Every human population seems to transgress against the laws of raw nourishment and beauty with no further regard to future consequences than experience has taught to be necessary. The limits of the indulgences are tested repeatedly and then moderated so as to make it difficult to ascertain what is leading to the demise. This moderated level of indulgence is then called "normal."

Through simple logic, we see that a brown bear is clearly more carnivorous than a human with its claws and teeth, and yet a brown bear eats a diet of 95-97% raw-plant-food. The longest-living Hunza people of northern Pakistan live on a diet containing less than 1% meat. Consider that between 1840 and 1974, the quantity of meat eaten per person in the United States increased five times. During roughly the same time, America went from the healthiest nation in world in 1900, out of 100 surveyed, to dead last in 1990. The direction we should all be moving is increasingly becoming more clear.

Of course, depending on each individual situation, room must be made for a transition away from animal products. Of all animal foods, young fish and game contain better quality oils and fats in their tissues in general. And these, if eaten at all, should be eaten sparingly. Eating meat and/or fish every day is not natural and is abusive to the planet's resources. If one is going to eat meat, one should eat smoked fish (*smoking the fish does*

not corrupt the fats and oils), young wild game (*with less palmitin and stearin*), and/or bone marrow (*an alkaline fat source similar in composition to olives*) to maintain a condition of eating for beauty.

Understand that everything we are physically made up of (*our teeth, skin, internal organs*) is composed of colloidal minerals. Colloidal minerals are living minerals suspended in a solution with energy. They are the foundational building blocks of life. These are the minerals found in living plant foods. Plants draw minerals from the soil and also create minerals, then suspend them with energy in the protoplasm of the leaf, fruit, flower or in other parts of their structure.

Now here is the interesting thing: whether we like it or love it, we are composed of concentrated plants. Every animal takes in plant food directly or indirectly and concentrates it. So, for example, a zebra is physically nothing more nor less than concentrated grass. And the lion that feeds on the zebra is also simply concentrated grass. There is nothing in the zebra that was not in the grass, and nothing in the lion that was not in the grass. A steak is actually concentrated grass (*devoid of alkaline minerals*)!

The American Dietetic Association (ADA), the world's largest organization of professional dieticians, published the following statement in 1988:

"There is a considerable amount of scientific research and figures to suggest the positive relation between a vegetarian lifestyle and the decrease of several different conditions and chronic degenerative diseases like obesity, heart/coronary disease, hypertension, diabetes mellitus, colon cancer, and others. Vegetarians also present the lowest percentages in osteoporosis, lung cancer, breast cancer, gallstone, kidney stone, and colon cancer.

Although vegetarian diets normally satisfy and some exceed the protein needs/requirements, they provide less protein than/compared to non-vegetarian diets. This lower intake/consumption in protein might be beneficial/good however, and is related/associated to a lower risk of osteoporosis and a noticeable improvement in the renal function (*kidney work*) in individuals with this problem...

The opinion of the American Dietetics Association regarding vegetarian diets is that they are healthy and nutritious/nutritionally adequate."

Once we know this, then the confusion about animal food is dispelled.

As we think about it clearly, we see that animals simply concentrate plant foods to form their tissues. And if there is toxicity in their air, water, and/or food environment — such as chemicals, pesticides, herbicides, larvicides, fungicides, detergents, bleaches, toxic solvents, etc. — then these toxins accumulate in the animal. I was surprised when I learned that dairy products contain five times as many pesticides as commercial fruits and vegetables. And flesh foods, such as fish or chicken, contain fifteen times as many pesticide residues as commercial fruits and vegetables! (See Gabriel Cousens' book *Conscious Eating* and John Robbins' *Diet For A New America*). Animals concentrate pollutants and store them in the center of their fat cells and in other areas of their bodies.

We do not live in the same world that existed 200 years ago. Pollution is rampant. Chemicals are everywhere. No source of tap water anywhere in world is safe to drink (*except in Iceland!*). People often ask me at my seminars, "Do you think I should get a filter for the tap water in my house?" I tell them, "You either get a filter or you become a filter!" Animal tissues accumulate toxicity from the environment — they filter it. Every animal eaten contains a megadose of toxicity. Ethical considerations aside, animal products are poor food choices.

Consider the wise words of the Greek philosopher Pythagorus:
"The land around us grows the most exquisite and delicious fruits in plenty. The Earth gives enough nourishment from just its vegetable realm, without the need for torture or violence."

When you eat raw-plant-foods and choose to move away from animal food for a considerable period of time, you become more alkaline and eventually reacquire your true sense of taste and smell; you feel a more wholesome, pure and exquisite enjoyment during meals.

Eating raw-plant-foods simplifies the whole eating process. It ends the need for reading packaging labels and hoping that one is not ingesting too many chemicals and toxins. You never know what you are getting with animal products and cooked and packaged foods. For example, piperonal (*found in ice cream*) is used instead of vanilla. It is also a chemical used to kill lice. When eating for beauty, one no longer has to worry about what steroids and drugs have been injected into the animal and dairy products, or the artificial colors or preservatives added to packaged foods.

Listen and Succeed

Because the present civilization feeds upon lifeless, indigestible materials, fast food, chemicals, drugs, and toxins of all descriptions, much of its art, architecture, cinema, music, literature, and sculpture are devoid of the raw essence of beauty. The façade of beauty is there, but the inner seeds are not. Inner toxicity has created the dismal corporate cities we see on the outside. We know that no other civilization has ever produced so much pollution and ugliness. Even in spite of all this, some artists and creators are still able to produce beautiful masterpieces. Yet this is difficult when one has been disconnected from mother nature and her infinite source of inspiration.

In essence, the message of this book is about how to make it easier to represent beauty in every manifestation. Society's dismal elements and disconnection can all be reversed right now, in a moment, through an inner transformation inspired by new knowledge.

I have come to deeply understand that knowledge is the only difference between someone who succeeds on a raw-plant-food approach and one who does not. This is both self-knowledge and learned knowledge. Continue the learning process in every facet of your life.

Raw-food nutrition is a frontier science and is always full of many startling secrets and surprises, many of which we will explore.

In any field, it is always best to listen only to those who are getting the results you desire. The transformation raw-food nutrition has brought into my life is visible for all to see. The authors of other diet books should be subject to public view in order to see who really walks their talk and whose diet really produces results.

I have been eating only raw-food since 1994. I have found this journey to be, by far, the most physically and spiritually beautifying experience of my life. The raw-food diet has helped me tap into more of my pure essence. It has created for me — and it can for you too — a new inner aliveness, glow, and charisma.

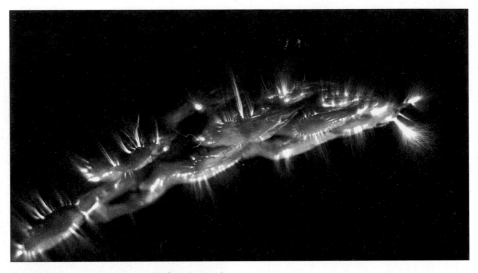

Cooked Organic Asparagus *(Kirlian Image)*

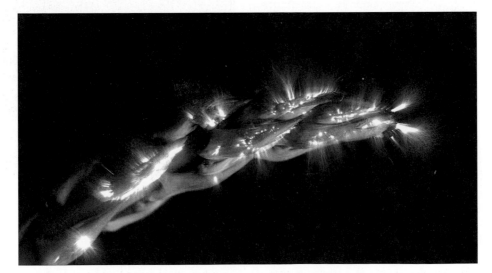

Raw Organic Asparagus *(Kirlian Image)*

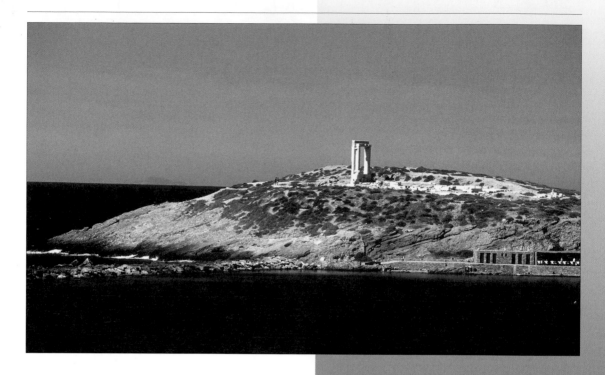

THE ACID/ALKALINE BALANCE SIMPLIFIED

Achieving that perfect balance depends predominantly on understanding and applying the acid/alkaline balance to your diet.

*T*he purpose of eating raw-foods is to lead you down a corridor so that you see doors that would not have opened to you previously, to allow your intuition and food instincts to become clearer, to move you from one opportunity to another *(from one synchronicity to another)* and to bring you into a more profound symmetry. All of these aspects become reality when one finds balance eating raw-foods — "balance" being the key word.

Achieving that perfect balance depends predominantly on understanding and applying the acid/alkaline balance to your diet.

Most nutritionists now agree that maintaining a balance of acidity and alkalinity in our bodily tissues is one of the primary roles of nutrition. This balance of acidity to alkalinity is usually referred to as pH *(per hydrogen)*. The acid/alkaline *(pH)* balance ranges from totally acid at 0.0 to totally alkaline at 14.0, with 7.0 being neutral. To a significant degree, the body uses electrolyte minerals to control pH. An electrolyte is a mineral that, in solution, conducts electricity. Sodium, potassium, calcium, magnesium, lithium, and phosphorus are the body's primary electrolytes.

Our ideal blood pH range is from 7.35 to 7.40. Other tissues in our bodies are more acidic, such as our muscles and skin *(6.8 pH)*. Ideally, our tissues overall, when added together and averaged, should be around 7.0 pH. Typically, we find that people who have eaten a standard diet all of their lives become unbalanced and acidic, and their overall net pH can drop to 6.3 or 6.2 or even lower.

Acidity is the underlying cause of all the ailments that mar beauty. Acidity creates inflammation, puffiness, asymmetry, and contraction of the tissues. The only way to correct this imbalance is to eat a ratio of foods that are more alkaline than acidic, and to get in the habit of drinking high quality spring water.

Every book on nutrition seems to have a different opinion on what foods are acidic and what foods are alkaline. The information in this chapter is designed to simplify that information into a usable system through which you can keep yourself in balance throughout all steps of your dietary transition and maintenance. The insight presented in this chapter is a common sense simplification that works. And you can prove it by experience and dispel for yourself many of the acid/alkaline myths.

The Role of Minerals

Ninety-five percent of the body's activities are run by minerals, not vitamins. Our biochemistry is mineral-dependent.

As has been mentioned previously, each cell contains over 4,000 enzymes. Every one of those enzymes is fully activated only when there are significant quantities of major and trace minerals present from eating the right diet.

Generally, the higher the concentration of minerals within a food, the better. Wild foods on average contain the most minerals. Homegrown and organic foods also contain a significant quantity of minerals as compared to commercial, chemically-grown foods. The beauty of our hair, skin, and nails depends on how mineralized we are. As you eat heavily mineralized raw-plant-food in

the right balance, you will become like a beautiful fruit tree firmly rooted in the earth with a deep and solid foundation.

The primary determinant of what foods are alkaline and what foods are acidic is the mineral content of the food.

Foods rich in alkaline minerals *(calcium, magnesium, silicon, iron, sodium, and manganese)* create alkalinity in the body.

Foods rich in acidic minerals *(phosphorus, chlorine, iodine, nitrogen, and to some degree sulfur)* create acidity in the body.

We need both alkaline- and acid-forming foods to be healthy and in balance. Acid-forming foods are not, in and of themselves, bad — they are simply acid-forming. An excess of acidity is, however, quite harmful over the short and long term as it leads to inflammation, contraction, stiffness, tissue degeneration, water retention, itchy skin, and more.

The Mineral Directive Principle

Minerals are built up in the different parts of a plant or animal based on some unknown directive principle. Some areas of the plant or animal get the acid-forming minerals, some areas get the alkaline-forming minerals. For example, mature wheat plants may contain up to 67% silica *(an alkaline-forming compound)*, and even as much as 87% silica in the husk. However, no silica is found in the grain seed. The grain seed contains a preponderance of phosphorous *(an acid-forming mineral)* in quantities far exceeding anything found in any other part of the plant. In comparing the straw to the husk to the grain seed, we find the compounds as described on the following page.

We also find that the amount of iron varies widely in different parts of the cabbage plant. For instance, the mature green leaves of cabbage contain four times as much iron as the inner leaves.

The Acid/Alkaline Chart is based on the mineral-directive principle. This principle

Straw		Husk		Grain Seed	
13.6%	K_2O (potassium, neutral)	9.1%	K_2O (potassium, neutral)	33.4%	K_2O (potassium, neutral)
1.4%	Na_2O (sodium, alkaline)	1.8%	Na_2O (sodium, alkaline)	3.2%	Na_2O (sodium, alkaline)
5.8%	CaO (calcium, alkaline)	1.9%	CaO (calcium, alkaline)	4.3%	CaO (calcium, alkaline)
2.0%	MgO (magnesium, alkaline)	1.3%	MgO (magnesium, alkaline)	12.0%	MgO (magnesium, alkaline)
0.6%	Fe_2O_3 (iron, alkaline)	0.4%	Fe_2O_3 (iron, alkaline)	2.2%	Fe_2O_3 (iron, alkaline)
4.8%	P_2O_5 (phosphorus, acidic)	4.3%	P_2O_5 (phosphorus, acidic)	44.0%	P_2O_5 (phosphorus, acidic)
2.4%	SO_3 (sulfur, acidic)	81.2%	SiO_2 (silicon, alkaline)		
67.5%	SiO_2 (silicon, alkaline)				

states that minerals are attracted to different areas of plants and animals. As the chart demonstrates, alkaline minerals are found in the leaves and stems of plants and in the bones of animals. Acidic minerals are found in the seeds and roots of plants and the muscles of animals. Fruits and flowers may be slightly acidic, slightly alkaline, or neutral. The organs and tissues of animals may be slightly acidic, slightly alkaline, or neutral.

How does this chart work? If one eats something acidic (such as a seed), then one should also eat something alkaline (green leaves). If an individual chooses to eat rice (seeds) for dinner, a nice green salad eaten along with that rice will make everything digest better as the acid/alkaline balance is met.

An understanding of this chart is what I call "primitive knowledge." This is

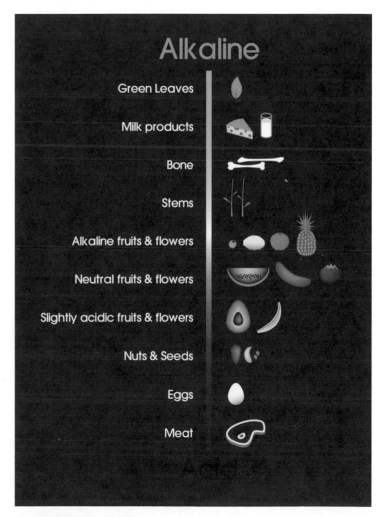

The Acid/Alkaline Chart

because "primitive" peoples all over the world appear to intuitively understand this balance.

From this chart we can begin to understand why civilization's diet is so acidic. Western civilization's diet consists mostly of roots, seeds, and animal muscles. This is translated into a burger *(the bun is seeds, the meat is a muscle)* and french fries *(roots)*. This is translated into a fancy steak *(muscle)*, potato *(root)* and peas *(seeds)*. The standard rice and beans dish is nothing more than seeds *(acid-forming)*.

When one has this awareness, it becomes easy to determine how lacking civilization's diet is in green-leafy foods. The only green-leafy food that is eaten seems to be commercial iceburg lettuce grown in mineral-deficient soils. To reverse an acidic condition, one should eat 1-2 organic green salads each day and drink a green vegetable juice and/or a juice containing a green superfood powder.

What we are looking for is a balance between acidity and alkalinity. Generally, most people are too acidic from eating the acid-forming "root, seed, muscle" diet throughout their lives. People in this category should eat more alkaline foods. Once a person has established a balance and can "feel" or "instinctively know" when one is too acidic or too alkaline, then it becomes important to eat acidic and alkaline foods in a balance to each other as needed. If you are not sure what your body needs, generally err on the side of eating more chlorophyll-rich green-leafy vegetables.

Many people have a prejudice against acidic foods. Remember, if a food is acidic, that is not a bad thing. We need to eat foods that are both acidic and alkaline — and we require these in a balance to each other. Neither is more important than the other. However, alkaline food is usually more important in the beginning years of changing our eating habits.

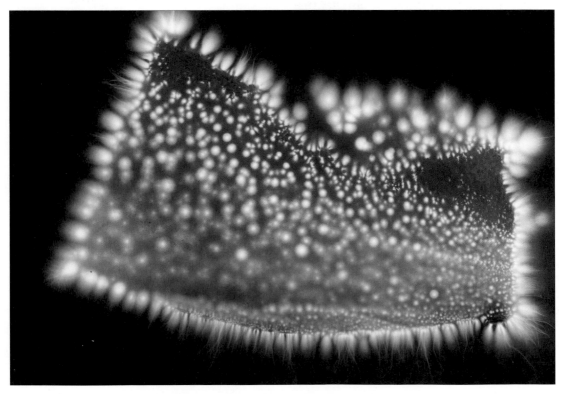

Organic Watermelon *(Kirlian Image)*
Watermelon rind is alkaline. The fleshy fruit is neutral in its effect on pH. The edible seeds are slightly acidic.

Acidity and Stimulants

Sure signs of acidity are a coffee habit, the desire to smoke cigarettes or marijuana, abuse of alcohol, cocaine use and/or other stronger legal or illegal drugs. These drugs contain alkaline stimulants *(sometimes called alkaloids)* that simulate the feeling of alkalinity and make one "high" for a while, before one comes back down. These drugs have a harsh edge to them. They deplete essential nutrients, exhaust the adrenal glands, and irritate and thicken the skin, lungs, and other organs. When one is acidic, then one may feel pleasantly relaxed or happy while taking these drugs. A major factor in overcoming these "addictions" is to create an acid/alkaline balance in the body. Once there is an acid/alkaline balance, then these drugs no longer make one high, but actually create a low.

Anybody who has ever taken drugs knows from experience how the high eventually becomes a low and the pleasure eventually becomes pain. Every addiction exists to cover up some emotional, spiritual, or physical discomfort or pain. Every addiction eventually reaches the point when the discomfort and pain can no longer be hidden and everything becomes more intense than ever. Eating green-leafy foods delivers to the body what it needs — vital alkalinity — and begins to displace addictive behavior.

Types of Foods and Their Acidity/Alkalinity
— Fruits —

A fruit is an edible product of a plant that contains the seed for reproduction. Certainly fruits are the most enchanting of all food groups. Fruits vary quite greatly in alkalinity and acidity. Based on the minerals they contain, some fruits are classified as alkaline while others are slightly acidic and some are neutral. Keep in mind that even the most acidic fruits are not as acidic as nuts, grains, or meat.

Alkaline Fruits

- Carob
- Olives
- Figs
- Papaya
- Pineapple
- Rambutan
- Grapefruit
- Lemon
- Lime
- Oranges
- Tangerines
- Citrus fruits
- Grapes *(with seeds)*
- Cherries
- Pomegranate
- Prickly Pear
- Wild Apples
- Hot Chiles
- Blackberry
- Raspberries
- Huckleberries
- Loganberries
- Passionfruit
- Cranberry
- Okra
- Barrel Cactus fruit
- Kiwi, etc.

Paradoxically, a typical characteristic of some alkaline fruits is that they contain a strong acidic compound, such as citric acid, that must be neutralized in order to extract and utilize the alkaline minerals.

Neutral Fruits

- Melons *(all types, including: Watermelon, Cantaloupe, Honeydew, Crenshaw, etc.)*
- Apples
- Bell Pepper
- Cucumber
- Tomato
- Mango
- Mangosteen
- Strawberries
- Blueberries
- Jackfruit
- Dragonfruit
- Apricots
- Peaches
- Nectarines
- Guava
- Persimmon *(with seeds)*
- Lychees
- Pumpkin
- Breadfruit
- Starfruit
- Noni
- Loquats
- Strawberry Guavas
- Milk fruit, etc.

Slightly Acidic Fruits

- Banana
- Avocado
- Cherimoya
- Durian
- Plums

- Dates
- Mulberry
- Sapote
- Mamey
- Persimmons *(without seeds)*

- Grapes *(without seeds)*
- Prunes
- Dried fruits *(except for figs)*

- Cacao
- Sugar Apples
- Soursop
- Akee, etc.

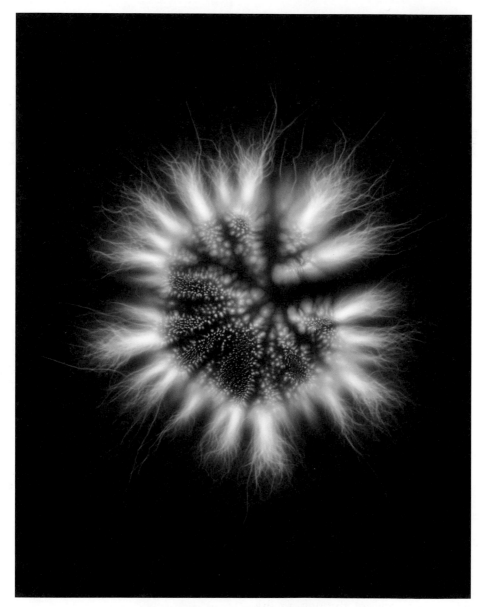

Malva: a common, wild green-leafy garden food (*Kirlian Image*)

— Flowers —

Flowers are a pleasant treat on any salad. They actually have quite amazing nutritional properties. The pollen of flowers, for example, is a high-grade protein containing many trace minerals. This is collected by bees and is usually available in health-food stores as bee pollen. Bee pollen is best eaten fresh. It goes rancid quickly. To test if bee pollen is rancid, place some into a bottle of water and shake vigorously. Then let the water and pollen sit. If the pollen sinks, it is good and fresh; if it floats, it is rancid.

We might take note that soaps and shampoos are often flower-scented, whereas we never hear of body-care products that are meat and cheese scented.

— Green-Leafy Vegetables —

Green-leafy vegetables are probably the most important group of foods. Green leaves are the best source of alkaline minerals, contain the best fiber, have many calming, anti-stress properties, and are the best source of chlorophyll. Chlorophyll is a blood-builder and one of nature's greatest healers. Green-leafy foods are the most abundant foods on earth. In July of 1940, a comprehensive report written by Dr. Benjamin Gurskin, director of experimental pathology at Temple University, focusing on 1,200 patients treated with chlorophyll was published in the *American Journal of Surgery*. On the power of chlorophyll, he said, "It is interesting to note there is not a single case recorded in which improvement or cure has not taken place." In 1950, Dr. Howard Westcott found that just 100 milligrams of chlorophyll in the diet neutralized bad breath, body odor, menstrual odors, and foul-smelling urine and stools.

— Root Vegetables —

These vary from neutral to acidic in nature. Radishes, onions and burdock root are the closest to neutral, while potatoes and carrots are more acidic.

The toxic compounds solanine and chaconine, known to be found in the eye of the potato, are actually present throughout the entire potato. A staple diet of potatoes robs vitamin A from the system. Because potatoes are extremely hybridized, they attract the attention of various fungi looking to "weed out the weak." Because of the prevalence of fungal breakouts in standard hybrid potatoes, they must be treated with large amounts of fungicides.

— Nuts & Seeds —

Nuts and seeds include all well-known nuts and seed varieties from macadamia nuts to pumpkin seeds, and everything in between. Grain and rice products also fall into the category of nuts and seeds. Thus, bread and pasta are seed products.

Nuts and seeds contain explosive phosphoric compounds that create the potential for quick growth of a young plant. All nuts and seeds are acidic in nature, with some being less acidic than others. Millet is definitely less acidic than wheat grain. Almonds are less acidic than walnuts or macadamia nuts.

Soaking nuts and seeds in water tends to deactivate acids and enzyme inhibitors *(enzyme inhibitors make nuts harder to digest)*. Thus soaked nuts and seeds are more alkaline, but they cannot be classified as truly alkaline until they sprout and grow green leaves.

The entire growth process of a nut or seed involves a conversion of phosphoric compounds into calcium, and sometimes silicon compounds *(such as in blades of grass in the mature state)*.

Coconut water is slightly alkaline if the coconuts are wild. Sweet coconut water from Thailand coconuts, found in many Asian markets and healthfood stores, is slightly acidic in its effect on the body. Coconut flesh is slightly acidic but not as acidic as other nuts and seeds.

— Grains —

Breads and other cooked grains, in general, are coarse foods. If one's metabolism primarily burns fat and/or protein as a fuel, starchy breads will cause excessive weight gain and puffiness in the face. If one primarily burns carbohydrate sugars as a fuel, then cooked fat/oil will cause weight gain and facial puffiness. Sprouted grain is a better option than cooked grain. Generally, sprouted mani-tok wild rice is the most digestible of the sprouted grains.

— Meat —

Meat denotes the muscle of an animal. This includes fish, pork, steak, chicken, beef, hamburger, duck, lamb, rabbit, goose, cornish hen, etc. Meat is built up of phosphoric compounds and is acidic in nature.

— Bone —

Bone marrow is an alkaline fat source — a relatively rare commodity in nature (olives are one of the only plant-based alkaline-fat sources).

If one is going to get an adequate acid/alkaline balance eating meat (muscle), one must eat the bone like the animals do, to get at the alkaline minerals there. This is the natural way of things, but is generally not recommended because the bone of factory-farmed animals contains sizeable percentages of toxins — including heavy metals, such as lead.

The problems with eating bone (possibility of choking, heavy metals, etc.) make it unsuitable to eat with the muscle. So, if one eats meat, one should also eat green-leafy vegetable salads to maintain an acid/alkaline balance.

Like other beings, we also store heavy metals in our bones. After eating living raw-foods for several months to a year it is not uncommon to see the levels of lead, cadmium, and other metals increase in the bloodstream. This is part of the body's cleansing process. This is because healthy minerals (such as calcium) displace heavy metals (such as lead) in the bone and bone marrow.

— Dairy Products —

This category includes the milk products of cows and goats (cheese, goat's cheese, whey, milk, kefir, yogurt, etc.). Based on their high alkaline mineral content, dairy products are alkaline if one can digest them. That is a big "if," because most people do not have the enzymes necessary to digest dairy products from cows. Cow's milk and cow cheeses are gluey, mucus-forming, and sticky — especially when pasteurized. Pasteurization destroys beneficial probiotic cultures (good bacteria) in the milk.

Yogurt is pasteurized and then cultured, so it does contain some probiotic cultures. Kefir is not pasteurized, thus, after it is cultured, it contains the best probiotic cultures of any dairy product.

A 12-year Harvard study of 78,000 women demonstrated that those who drink cow's milk are more likely to have osteoporosis and brittle bones (please read "Milk, Dietary Calcium and Bone Fractures In Women: A 12-Year Prospective Study" published in The American Journal of Public Health (1997;87:992-7) written by Feskanich, D., Willett, W.C., Stampfer, M.J., Colditz, G.A.). The countries that consume the most cow's milk have the highest rates of osteoporosis (Finland, United States and Canada). Please read John Robbins' books Diet For A New America and The Food Revolution for more information on this subject.

Enzymes are required in order to overcome and break down the thick, gluey structure of cow's milk and extract the minerals.

Unpasteurized goat's milk, goat cheese, and goat kefir are the best of the dairy products. They are much easier to digest, contain a high quantity of alkaline minerals, and are closer to human milk in composition.

— Eggs —

Eggs from chickens or other animals fit into the classification of "seeds." When eaten raw, egg whites (not yolks) contain strong enzyme inhibitors. This means they require internal enzymes from the pancreas to digest. It also means they tax the body if eaten excessively. These enzyme inhibitors are destroyed by cooking. Raw egg yolks contain highly-nutritious lecithin, which is destroyed by cooking. Eggs, like seeds, are acid-forming.

— Soda/Pop —

Soda is by far the most acid-forming of all foods. Soda is not really a food or drink at all, but a collection of acidic chemicals (*carbonic acid, phosphoric acid, etc.*). One eight-ounce glass of soda is so acid-forming that it requires 30 eight-ounce glasses of water to dilute it and normalize the pH. There is no radiance or majesty in the acid-chemical soup called soda. Soda demineralizes the bones, teeth, and skin.

Other Elements of The Acid/Alkaline Balance

Alkaline - Foods rich in alkaline minerals.	**Acid - Foods rich in acidic minerals.**
• Faith	• Worry
• Hope	• Stress
• Friendship	• Hatred
• Chlorophyll	• Sugar
• Love	• Fear
• Green juice	• Alcohol
• Spring water at the source	• Tap water
• Laughter	• Anger
• Deep breathing	• Shallow breathing
• Medicinal herbs	• Drugs, chemicals, or toxins.

Symptoms of Being Too Acidic:

- Tense muscles
- Stress headaches
- Anger
- Short temper
- Chronic negative thoughts
- Addictions to coffee, cigarettes, smoking marijuana, cocaine, crystal meth-amphetamine, ecstasy, etc.
- Itchy skin
- Acne

Symptoms of Being Too Alkaline:

- Laziness
- Spaciness
- Lack of drive
- Excessively passive
- Feelings of being too cold
- Weakness

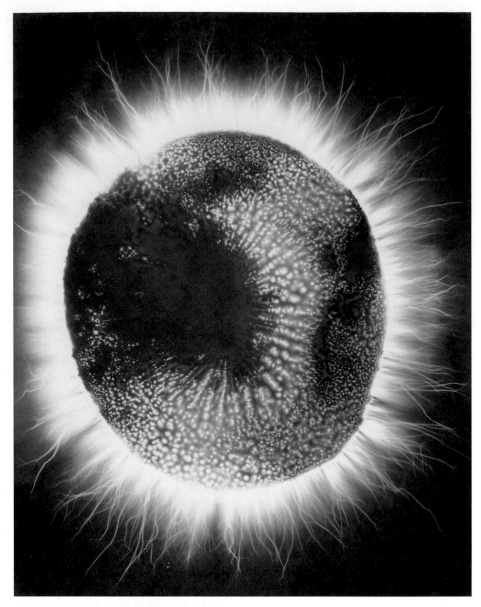

Organic Kiwi (*Kirlian Image)*

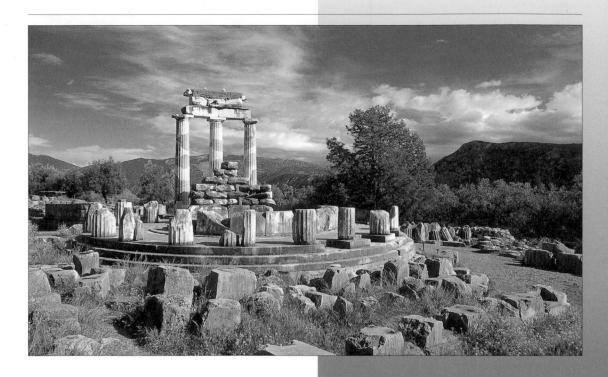

General wisdom dictates that there are three components to the human diet — proteins, carbohydrates, and fats. Proteins *(made up of amino acids)* contain the basic building materials of the body and are most useful when found in uncooked plant foods. All the strongest, largest animals on the Earth feed their muscles and enormous bodies with plants — especially green leaves and algae. Carbohydrates *(sugars)* are sources of quick energy and are best derived from mineral-rich sweet fruits. Fats consist of solid or liquid oils that lubricate the intestines and joints, and are sources of long-term energy. Fat is best derived from such foods as avocados, olives, olive oil, nuts, many seeds, seed oils, and the durian fruit.

Fats, carbohydrates, and proteins form the necessary elements of the human diet. This means that each of these food classes must be present in some significant percentage in the diet. The percentage for each class varies from person to person depending on their metabolic type, current state of digestion, health history, health goals, etc. Some people, like myself, burn dietary fats as their primary fuel. This could mean 60% of my diet on any given day consists of fats. Others primarily burn carbohydrates as a fuel. This might mean that 60% of their diet consists of carbohydrates. Others, though usually a smaller percentage, might burn protein *(amino acids)* as their primary fuel.

Proteins, carbohydrates, and fats form the points of a triangle. The goal is to stay balanced within the triangle.

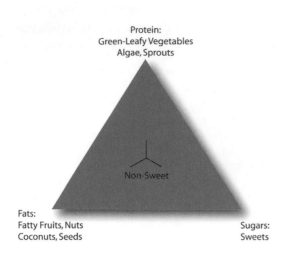

Protein:
Green-Leafy Vegetables
Algae, Sprouts

Non-Sweet

Fats:
Fatty Fruits, Nuts
Coconuts, Seeds

Sugars:
Sweets

Let's look at the different food classes and their roles:

Fats

Plant fats contain many oils that are favorable to our appearance. Avocados, olives, raw nuts, certain raw seeds, young coconuts, and the Southeast Asian fruit called durian have impressive youthening qualities.

Many plant fats are cold-pressed to create wonderful oils such as olive oil, hemp oil, borage seed oil, primrose oil, flax-seed oil, etc. Cold-pressed oils retain more sensitive elements and delicate flavors than heat-processed oils.

Dr. Weston Price was a dentist who studied the beautiful teeth of people raised on traditional diets, as compared to the poor teeth of those raised on the demineralized foods of civilization. Based on his findings, Dr. Price authored the classic nutrition text, *Nutrition and Physical Degeneration*. He discovered that fat-soluble vitamins found in raw fats/oils promoted the beautiful bone structure, wide palate, flawless well-spaced teeth, and handsome, well-proportioned faces that characterized members of isolated traditional cultures.

Raw or cold-pressed fats and oils are one of the best foods to include in our diet because they beautify the skin, lubricate the joints and intestines, strengthen cell membranes, and restore fat-soluble nutrients to the tissues.

There is a dramatic difference between raw fats/oils and cooked fats/oils.

Cooked fats/oils are not miscible with water. Since we are a water-based life-form, this presents a challenge to the digestive system and liver. Cooked fats/oils tend to be broken down improperly. They lead to acne, skin disorders, liver stagnation, porous cell membranes, body odor, and nutritional deficiencies. Cooked fats/oils are fattening and lead to many health challenges. That is why we hear unfavorable reports about fats/oils in the media and in science journals.

Closer inspection reveals that animal foods advertised as being supposedly low in fat are still high in fat. Consider that lean ground beef provides about 54% of its calories in the form of fat. 51% of the calories from chicken comes from fat, as do 40% of the calories of salmon. The best way to avoid a high cooked-fat diet is to abstain from all cooked foods and animal products.

The quantity of raw fats/oils eaten should be within the limit of what an individual can handle based on their metabolism. As an example: for some, half an avocado per day is as much as can be handled; for others, two to three avocados a day is healthy. Generally, it is a good rule to eat fats (*especially raw nuts and seeds*) with green-leafy salads for ease of digestion. The excessive intake of fats/oils, even if it is raw fat/oils, can lead to facial pimples and a general feeling of lethargy.

The spicy sulfurous elements found in hot peppers, onions, garlic, arugula, radishes, and watercress can be "cooled" or "cut" by eating fats such as avocados, macadamia nuts, olives, olive oil, and coconut oil. Fats help digest spicy sulfur compounds. The opposite is also true: spicy sulfur compounds help digest fats. Sulfur compounds cause fat to disperse in the bloodstream, preventing the fat from clumping (*agglutinating*) in the blood.

— Types of Fats —

The arrangement of hydrogen determines if a fat is saturated, monounsaturated, or polyunsaturated. The more hydrogen that is present *(in the fat)*, the more saturated the fat.

The best saturated fats include cold-pressed coconut oil *(sometimes called coconut butter)* and cold-pressed palm kernel oil.

The best monounsaturated fats include avocados, olives, raw nuts *(except polyunsaturated walnuts)*, stone-crushed olive oil, and durian.

The best polyunsaturated fats include hemp oil, hemp seeds, primrose oil, borage seed oil, flax, flax oil, walnuts.

Excellent Choices for Dietary Fat

Fruits

- Avocado
- Durian
- Olives
- Stone-crushed olive oil

Nuts

- Raw nuts of all kinds and raw nut butters

Seeds

- Pumpkin seeds or raw pumpkin seed butter
- Sesame seeds or raw black tahini
- Sunflower seeds or raw sunflower butter
- Hemp seeds
- Flax seeds
- Seed oils *(cold-pressed)*
- Young coconuts
- Coconut butter/oil

Carbohydrates (Sugars)

The best source of carbohydrates is organic fruits or wild fruits that contain seeds. Organic and/or wild fruits sold at natural food stores and farmer's markets always contain more minerals than commercially-grown varieties sold at supermarkets. Generally, the richer a sweet fruit is in minerals, the better. Mineral content is usually detectable in fruit quality, flavor, texture, and the overall richness of the fruit.

Fruits contain simple sugars such as glucose and fructose. These sugars act as fuel for the body. Simple sugars are used by each cell's power-station — the mitochondria. The mitochondria create nucleotides *(ATP, GTP)* which, in turn, fuel the inside of the cell. Some people require more operational fuel than others depending on their metabolism and how much they exercise *(more exercise requires more fuel/fruit)*.

Often we find that the term "carbohydrate" is a fancy way of saying cooked sugar and/or starch. This term is frequently used to mask the quantity of sugar and starch found in such foods as bread, pasta, rice, rice cakes, baked potatoes, potato chips, corn chips, high fructose corn syrup, soy milk, alcohol, soda, seedless fruits, etc. All of these foods are derived from wheat seeds, barley seeds, soy beans, corn, beets, potatoes, and tree grafting processes. These long-domesticated, chemically-grown, hybridized crops are high in carbohydrates, energetically weak, and low in minerals.

Foods that have the characteristic of being high in sugar *(carbohydrates)* and low in minerals contribute to an increase of mold and fungus *(candida)* in the body, causing lethargy and laziness. Mold and fungus are nature's recyclers; they are always trying to weed out the weak plants. Mold and fungus find favorable growing environments in those who eat the weak crops described above.

The most weakening of all foods and drinks is soda or cola. Soda is not even a food, but rather, it is a strange mixture of chemicals and sugar *(or artificial sugar)*. Soda has no relationship with anything natural.

Weak foods that are high in carbohydrates and low in minerals have an inflammatory, irritating effect on our tissues. They lead us step-by-step toward addictive relationships with foods *(notice how addictive these foods can be)*. And then, eventually, they create conditions of hypoglycemia and sugar diabetes.

Sugar diabetes, sometimes called diabetes mellitus, is one of the most common diseases of the modern age. Mellitus is a combination of two Latin words: "mel," which in Latin is honey, and "itis" for inflammation. People with sugar diabetes have a lifespan 1/3 shorter than nondiabetics.

In terms of outward appearance, the abuse of cooked carbohydrate foods makes the skin pale-white and often puffy. Internally, carbohydrate abuse steadily robs the pancreas, adrenals, and bones of vital minerals. It diminishes the effectiveness of the immune system.

— Refined Sugar —

Heroin is produced by taking the juice of certain poppy varieties and refining it into opium, then morphine, and finally into heroin. Similarly, refined sugar is produced from taking the juice of sugar cane or beet and refining it into molasses, then brown sugar, and finally into white sugar.

The beet was first hybridized (bred for sweetness) and processed into sugar by the Frenchman Benjamin Delessert in 1812. Napoleon awarded him the Legion of Honor and ordered beets to be planted everywhere in France in order to facilitate the ever-growing desire for refined sugar.

Refined sugar is a drug that causes artificial highs, mood swings, depression, and energy crashes. In the 16th century, refined sugar was considered and used as a recreational drug in the royal courts of Europe.

It takes 1.1 kilograms (2.5 pounds) of sugar beets to create a mere 0.14 kilograms (5 ounces) of refined sugar. It is 8 times as concentrated as flour. Refined sugar is essentially a concentrated, crystallized acid.

Refined sugar (chemically in the form of sucrose) is close in chemical composition to glucose, so it largely escapes processing by the liver. When one ingests it, the sucrose passes into the blood, where the glucose level has already been established in precise balance with oxygen. The blood sugar level is thus drastically increased.

Consuming refined sugar leaches precious minerals (chromium, zinc, sulfur, vanadium, calcium) from the body due to the demands it makes on insulin production and the blood sugar system. When refined sugar is ingested every day, especially by someone who is becoming more and more demineralized, it eventually produces an increasingly acidic condition and more alkaline minerals are required from the bones to buffer or neutralize the situation. This eventually leads to spongy, weak bones (osteoporosis).

Carbohydrates are metabolized with the help of B vitamins. More B vitamins are needed for those who take in a large amount of carbohydrates. Refined sugar has the habit of robbing the body of precious B vitamins, which help the body deal with stress. A lack of B vitamins can cause chapped lips and wrinkles.

Refined sugar is especially damaging to the skin because it attaches to collagen molecules in the skin, causing cross-linking, stiffness, and inflexibility. I have also seen these collagen-damaging effects in some people who eat excessive amounts of fruit (especially seedless fruit) and/or carrot juice (which is extremely high in sugar). Age and liver spots on the skin are created when sugar and collagen react repeatedly over time, causing what is known scientifically as a Browning reaction.

I am not suggesting that you should diminish or control your intake of refined sugar (sometimes called high fructose corn syrup). I am suggesting that you should completely eliminate all refined sugar from your diet. Use honey, raw agave cactus nectar, yacon root syrup, stevia, dried figs, or other dried fruits as sweeteners in the initial stage of dietary transition.

— Understanding —
The Yin/Yang Balance

According to Oriental philosophy, everything in nature follows a yin/yang balance, including dietary patterns. Sugar is the extreme yin food and red meat is the extreme yang food. These are two ends of a see-saw! Visualize refined sugar on one side, red meat on the other. Even though they are both toxic foods, together they will actually balance each other out in terms of the way they stimulate a person. If one is eliminated without the other, the see-saw will swing out of balance. Both must be removed from the diet at the same time. This is a key understanding in transitioning your diet.

In countries where meat, and red meat in particular, is rarely eaten, and where the diet is centered on rice *(a carbohydrate)*, there is no balance to the see-saw effect created by refined sugar. This is why refined sugar has caused even more trouble in Asia than anywhere else in the world.

— Improving Carbohydrate Choices —
Improving the quality of your carbohydrates improves the quality of your health and life. Eliminating refined sugar and white flour, then replacing those with whole foods and natural fruits *(with seeds)* is the core of any sensible diet.

The best choice is to select foods that are richly mineralized and are medium to low in sugar. Certainly organic, homegrown, and/or wild fruits with seeds are excellent choices because they are always higher in minerals than the type of commercially-grown fruits found in most supermarkets.

In terms of cooked foods, yams and sweet potatoes are a far better choice than regular potatoes because they contain half the sugar and twice the minerals as regular potatoes.

Protein
Proteins are molecular compounds that are integral to the life functions of every type of living cell. These large, complex molecules might contain as many as a thousand amino acid units. Of the 22 amino acids, only a few will be found in most proteins. The variance in the total number of amino acids present and the order of amino acids in the chain accounts for the vast number of different types of protein.

Most of the flesh in animals and most of the organic material in plants are proteins. All enzymes, antigens, antibodies, and hormones are proteins.

Excellent Carbohydrate Choices

Raw
- Agave cactus nectar
  (sap from the agave plant)
- Apples
- Berries of all kinds
- Cacao fruit
- Cherimoyas
  (includes atemoyas, sugar apples, paw-paws, and another 60 fruits in this class)
- Citrus fruits with seeds
- Dragonfruit
- Durian
- Figs
- Grapes
- Jackfruit
- Mamey sapotes
- Mangos
- Mangosteen
- Melons of all kinds
  (if they contain seeds)
- Papayas
- Pears
- Sapotes
- Stone fruits
  (apricots, nectarines, peaches, plums)
- Yacon root syrup
- Young Thai coconut water
  (excellent to mix with green superfood powders such as Sun Is Shining Superfood)

Cooked Choices
- Ancient grain breads
  (kamut, spelt, wild rice)
- Breadfruit
- Sweet potatoes
- Yams
- Yucca Root

All protein contains the elements hydrogen, carbon, oxygen and especially nitrogen, although some contain phosphorous and sulfur as well.

Living cells use proteins (*amino acids*) as chemical building blocks for growth, repair, development, and a host of other vital tasks. In essence, it is amino acids that build muscle, strengthen tissues, repair cells, and maintain the structural integrity of the body.

Amino acids are essential in the formation of the two essential brain hormones: serotonin and dopamine, which play a strong role in how we feel each day.

Research has shown that the complementary protein principle, the idea that foods such as beans could be eaten with foods such as rice to create a complete protein, has been proven unnecessary as the body pools amino acids and can use them to create proteins even when certain amino acids are absent from the diet for a meal, a day, a week, etc.

Beans and legumes contain coarse proteins that are unfavorable for beauty. To some degree sprouted grain also contains coarse proteins that, when excessively eaten, disfavor beauty (*see Appendix B*).

Nuts are notoriously acid-forming and, as we have seen in the previous chapter, must be balanced by eating sufficient green-leafy vegetables.

In terms of protein, cooked animal protein is actually a poor-quality source of protein. It is coagulated, difficult to digest, creates inflammation in the tissues, and is rough on the kidneys. The elastic, light-weight polypeptides (*free-form amino acids*) found in plant foods make them a superior and ideal source of protein-building blocks.

If you are new to eating raw-foods, or simply new to dietary changes in general, I recommend that you include more proteins (*amino acids*) in your diet in the form of some of the protein-rich foods in the following list.

The Best Protein Foods

- Almonds
- Bee pollen
  (*probably the best of all high-protein foods*)
- Blue-green algae (from Klamath Lake)
- Brewer's yeast
  (*not good for those with candida or other fungal conditions in or outside the body*)
- Chlorella
- Durian
- Earth's Essential Elements
  (*E3 Live fresh algae*)
- Goji berries
  (*14% protein*)
- Grass powders
  (*dehydrated and powdered grasses*)
- Green-leafy vegetables
  (*such as parsley, spinach, kale, collards, green cabbage, arugula, etc.*)
- Hemp seeds
  (*contain the globular complete protein edestin*)
- Hemp protein
  (*30 grams of protein per tablespoon!*)
- Incan berries
  (*16% protein*)
- Maca
  (*powdered root superfood from the Andes*)
- Mature grasses
  (*chew on the blades before they have flowered*)
- Olives
- Propolis
  (*a resinous substance from saps collected by bees to help build the hive*)
- Pumpkin seeds
- Pure Synergy or Sun Is Shining Superfood
- Spirulina
- Sprouted grains
- Sprouted wild rice
- Sprouts of all types
- Vegetable powders
  (*dehydrated and powdered green vegetables*)

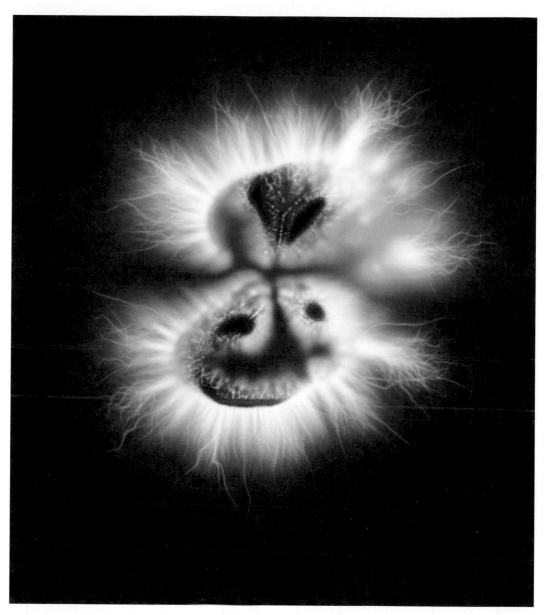

A Protein-Rich Buckwheat Sprout — viewed from above *(Kirlian Image)*

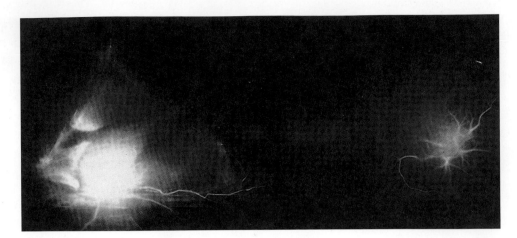

Olive oil on the left vs. Lard on the right *(Kirlian Image)*

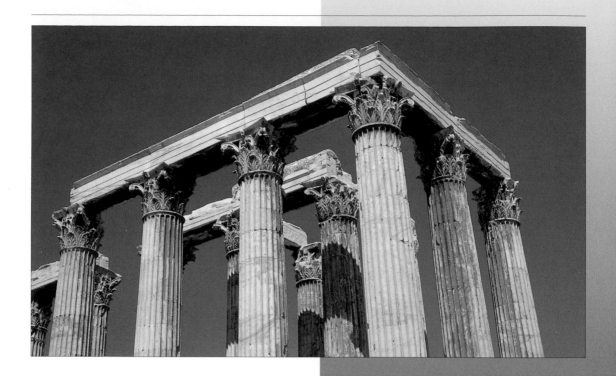

ELEMENTS OF THE BEAUTY DIET®

"Internal Cleanliness Creates External Beauty"

Certain factors are critically important in maintaining internal cleanliness. These factors help one to maintain and to thrive on a raw-food regimen. In this chapter we will cover the essential elements of The Beauty Diet® not already covered.

Proceed At Your Own Pace

The first element of The Beauty Diet® is to transition your body onto a living-plant-food diet at your own pace. The best strategy with which to do this is to proceed by stepping out of your comfort zone, but not into your shock zone. This means that you should do enough to stretch your mind, body, and spirit while at the same time staying within a reasonable boundary. For example, for those who are new to raw-foods, one may try to eat raw-food only throughout the day and have a cooked meal in the evening. *(Just doing this alone creates amazing positive results!).* For those who are already eating all raw-foods, fasting one day per week on juice or water may be an appropriate next step.

Remember: nutrition is an art — it is an art form. Every bite is a brush stroke. Every swallow is a new color. Each meal is a cloud or a tree or a flower — a piece of the painting that you are becoming. You are becoming an ever more attractive work of art. You are a work of art in progress.

Simplify. Keep everything fun and simple. As with anything, practice, experience, and rebound from challenges appropriately. Enjoy every step along the path toward perfect nutrition.

Water

Water is a universal solvent. We are a water-based lifeform. Water carries nutrients to every cell in our bodies. Water flushes out every toxin. Water alone can dissolve and wash away almost any impurity.

The first step in getting the body chemistry in proper order is to become well hydrated.

Nearly the entire population is suffering from chronic dehydration. Dr. Batmanghelidj's insightful book *Your Body's Many Cries For Water* makes this point clear. Dr. Batmanghelidj explains that all types of pains, obesity, and premature physical degeneration are related to being chronically dehydrated.

Being well hydrated increases the strength of our immune systems. Proper hydration keeps our skin and organs healthy. Hydration is essential in keeping us clear, bright, and beautiful. Hydration is the main factor that keeps one's tissues "juicy."

In this age, the challenge with water is its cleanliness. Most tap water is loaded with heavy metals, chlorine, fluoride, and microorganisms. Many of the river systems throughout the world are polluted and unfit to drink from, swim in, and/or eat things out of. There is only one place in the world where tap water is drinkable and that is in Iceland, where all tap water is natural spring water.

Fresh spring water — at the source — is the ideal water for human consumption. Spring water is the quintessential product of the Earth's natural hydrological cycle. Spring water bottled in glass is a great choice for drinking water.

Well water may be a great source of water, but it is being pulled up prematurely, before the water is ripe. Therefore it may actually contain too many sedimentary minerals such as iron or calcium. I recommend, for most well water sources, that they are filtered using a reverse osmosis water purification system before they are consumed.

Distilled water may be a reasonable drinking water choice (*for those living in cities*) if it is packaged in glass and "charged" before drinking (*for more on charging water, see below*). Distilled water in plastic containers should be avoided because the plastic leaches into the water (*this is often detectable by taste*). Plastic is detrimental because it mimics hormones in our bodies, causing glandular imbalances.

— Charging Water —

Charging water means giving a "life-pattern" or structure to the water at a microscopic level. The hydrogen molecules in water are closer together if the water is charged. This makes the water more polar (*strongly electrical*).

Adding a few pinches of Celtic Grey Mineral Sea Salt or Himalayan Pink Salt is a great way to charge water. These are some of the best choices for non-vegetable sources of salt. These salts each contain over eighty different minerals in similar ratios as they appear in sea water. They are "raw" salts, thus they differ from coagulated table salt and most "kiln-dried" sea salts that have had their minerals oxidized away through heating.

Other ways to charge water include adding MSM powder crystals (*more information on MSM is provided in Lesson 7*). At my office, we have distilled water delivered in glass. We have placed several quartz crystals in the distilled water dispenser, which charges the water, as has been proven with Kirlian photography.

Squeezing fruit juices or placing leaves of plants into water adds a charge. Squeezing lemons and/or limes into your water is an excellent choice because they have incredible cleansing and mucus-dissolving properties.

Putting water under full moonlight charges the water as well. Running water through a vortex (*the tornado effect*) improves its quality. Dr. Emoto has shown in his books *The Message from Water (volumes 1-3)*, that water responds to loving thoughts and even words written on a water bottle. Some believe that praying over your water before drinking it is also helpful. Water quality seems to always reflect our actions and intentions.

— How Much Water To Drink? —

We should ideally drink when our stomach is empty of food. Drinking water with food can dilute digestive fluids leading to poor absorption and constipation. The best time to drink water is upon rising in the morning. Drink at least 1/2 liter *(16 fluid ounces)* or more at that time.

The typical recommendation to drink "8-10 twelve-ounce glasses of water" each day is excessive if one eats 80%+ juicy raw-plant-foods. Even if one eats 100% raw-foods, however, drinking water each day is still very important. Plain water has its own flushing abilities that simply are not found in coconut water, fruits, and vegetable juices.

If one eats 80%+ raw-foods, I recommend drinking enough water based on the following ratio: Your total weight *(in pounds)* divided by 4 = # *(in ounces of water you should drink daily)*.

Take one's total weight *(in pounds)* and divide it by four. This will give a number. This number is then the number of fluid ounces of water one should drink in a day. For example, I weigh 170 pounds. I eat 100% raw-foods. 170 divided by 4 is 42.5. A good daily intake of water for me is 42.5 ounces *(this is a little more than a 32-ounce quart)*. *(One fluid ounce is equivalent to approximately 30 milliliters)*.

Be aware that dehydration can happen rapidly. An hour of intense exercise can cause you to lose a quart *(liter)* of water. A four-hour airline flight can cause you to lose up to a quart *(liter)* of water.

Building Hydrochloric Acid

When switching over to a diet containing more vegetables, it is important to build up hydrochloric acid in the stomach. Hydrochloric acid (HCl) is used by the stomach to break down fiber and plant roughage.

Over one's lifetime, the eating of animal foods, demineralized foods, and a few token

vegetables *(coupled with emotional stress)*, causes the body to lose its ability to produce HCl.

Protein-heavy animal products do not require HCl as it is not used to break down heavy proteins. Rather, it is used to tear apart plant fiber and roughage.

A lack of natural salts and vegetables in the diet and/or eating high quantities of "complex carbohydrates," and sugars *(which flush mineral salts from the body)* eventually causes the body to become deficient in chloride and, subsequently, in HCl. Even eating only fruit for several months can have this effect.

HCl is one of the body's first lines of defense, because it also destroys parasites, mold, harmful bacteria, and viruses. HCl activates pepsin; encourages the flow of bile and pancreatic enzymes; and facilitates absorption of nutrients, including folic acid, ascorbic acid, beta-carotene, plant-based *(non-heme)* iron, and some forms of calcium, magnesium, and zinc.

HCl is incapable of destroying proteins. Therefore enzymes *(since they are made of protein)* are unaffected by the presence of HCl in the stomach.

When HCl production is low, it affects the metabolism. It causes incomplete digestion of food and failure of assimilation. Common symptoms associated with low hydrochloric acid afflict a large portion of the population. They include:

- Allergies
- Adrenal exhaustion
- Anemia
- Bloating
- Brittle nails
- Candida
- Chronic fatigue syndrome
- Constipation
- Dry skin
- Gall stones
- Gastro-intestinal (GI) infections *(i.e. ulcers)*

- Hypoglycemia
- Inability to digest vegetables
- Lupus
- Mineral deficiencies
- Osteoporosis
- Parasites
- Protruding belly
- Rheumatoid arthritis
- Vitiligo
  (loss of skin pigmentation)
- Voracious appetite

Those who have studied nutrition may notice that symptoms of low HCl are similar to those of a fungal overgrowth in the body *(candida)* and a digestive enzyme deficiency. My experience is that low HCl, an internal fungal overgrowth and a digestive enzyme deficiency are nearly always found together.

How To Produce More Hydrochloric Acid

The body builds HCl out of salts. Natural salts found in salty vegetables restore HCl. Heavy salts, such as table salt or "kiln-dried" sea salt may be usable when one is young, but as vital energy decreases with age, they become difficult for the body to use to create HCl.

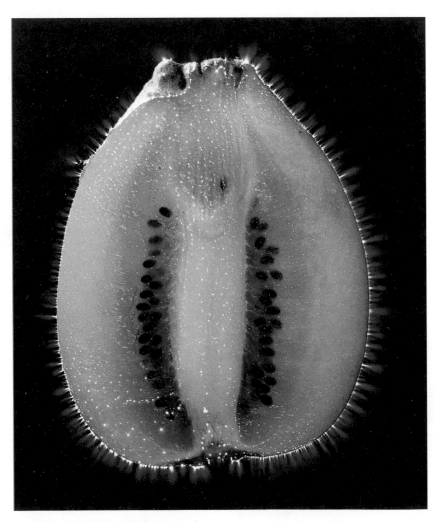

Raw Commercial Kiwi *(Kirlian Image)*

Excellent Foods and Vegetable Juices To Build Hydrochloric Acid

- Celery juice
- Spinach juice
- Chard juice
- Kale juice
- Lemon juice
  (before or with a salad)
- Raw apple cider vinegar
  (before or with a salad)
- Ginger juice
- Any vegetable juices that are rich in mineral salts *(salty to the taste)*
- Olives
  (not green)
- Celtic Grey Mineral Sea Salt or Himalayan Pink Salt
- Grass powders
- Sun Is Shining
  (a superfood blend and an excellent source of minerals)

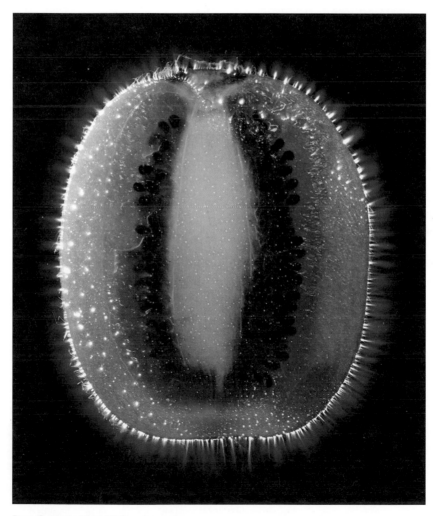

Raw Organic Kiwi *(Kirlian Image)*

Acidic foods can also help stimulate HCl production. Take a shot of lemon juice or raw apple cider vinegar to increase HCl production before eating a salad. A shot of ginger juice works effectively as well. Also, eating oranges or other citrus before, during, or after a salad may also be helpful for some people.

Certain herbs are helpful in building HCl as well. These include: herbal bitters, such as gentian or wormwood, and herbal stimulants, such as pepper or cayenne.

Betaine hydrochloride is an excellent supplement for increasing acids in the stomach to help break down food.

Kirlian Image

In Kirlian images organic foods show noticeably more luminescence.

Minerals are required as internal food-mineral cosmetics that add color and hue to the face, skin, hair, and nails. The more mineral density a food possesses, the less likely one is to overeat it. Eating mineral-deficient foods causes overeating because the body never finds what it is really looking for in food — minerals! Overeating and obesity both have an underlying physiological component — the search for minerals.

During the 1940s, Professor William Albrecht, one of the world's greatest soil scientists, then at the University of Missouri, analyzed 70,000 U.S. Navy dental records as a function of where in the U.S. the sailors were born and raised. His conclusion was that the health of the soil is the health of our bodies. The sailors from the topsoil-rich Midwest had far fewer dental cavities than sailors from other parts of the U.S. where the soil was more eroded and less rich in nutrients.

In 1993, Doctor's Data Lab of Chicago did a study published in the *Journal of Applied Nutrition (Vol. 45, Issue #1)*. For over two years, researchers collected foods, such as apples, corn, peas, and potatoes from organic food stores and regular supermarkets in the Chicago area, just like a typical shopper. Their lab test results showed that, by weight, organic produce contained at least twice the nutritional mineral content of regular supermarket produce and far less dangerous heavy-metal residues, such as aluminum, lead, and mercury.

Agriculture itself leads to deficiencies because croplands are typically improperly farmed and become mineral deficient. In the present era, hybridized or genetically-altered inferior seeds are used to grow plants that are weak, need to be heavily fertilized, and are

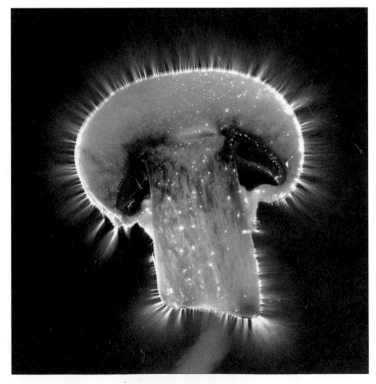

Raw Commercial Mushroom *(Kirlian Image)*

protected from natural selection by the use of pesticides. This is how most commercial foods are grown these days. These foods do not have enough minerals, life-force, or nutrients to maintain excellent health.

On March 9, 1993, *The New York Times* reported that 68 pesticide ingredients have been determined to cause cancer. The National Academy of Sciences released a finding that was written in *The USA Today* on June 28, 1993, which stated, "By the time the average child is a year old, s/he will have received the acceptable lifetime doses of 8 pesticides from 20 commonly eaten foods." Pesticides are unacceptable at any level, and definitely should be avoided on our food.

Organic food is not only grown without chemical pesticides, but it also contains more minerals than commercial food. In my experience, it is worth paying three to four times as much money for organic food than for chemically-grown food. It is better to pay more for something, than less for nothing. If we pay less now, we usually pay more later.

Every dollar we spend is actually a vote for the future. Every time we purchase organic food we support organic farmers, sustainable farming, and a sustainable future for all life on the planet. Pesticides are poisons and should never be used on anything.

One must definitely eat organic foods or better *(such as home-grown or wild foods)* in order to get enough quality minerals in the diet. If you owned a Rolls Royce, would you put poor-quality fuel in the gasoline tank? With an investment like that you would spend the extra money to get the best quality fuel you could find. Now your body is certainly worth more than a Rolls Royce! Quality food counts.

If you live in an area where organically-grown foods are scarce, mail order foods are available to you. The organization Sunfood Nutrition (www.sunfood.com) distributes bulk organic nuts, dried fruits, olives, stone-crushed olive oil, coconut oil, raw superfoods, and other items all over the world.

Homegrown Food

Nothing tastes better than a homegrown tomato — everybody knows that. Homegrown parsley, lettuce, cucumbers, and fruits of all kinds are just fantastic. If you do not have a garden, start one or ask to use part of a friend's or a community garden. If you do not have a yard, start a sprout garden in your kitchen. Have a look at Dr. Ann Wigmore's and Steve "The Sproutman" Meyerowitz's books on how to grow an indoor sprout garden.

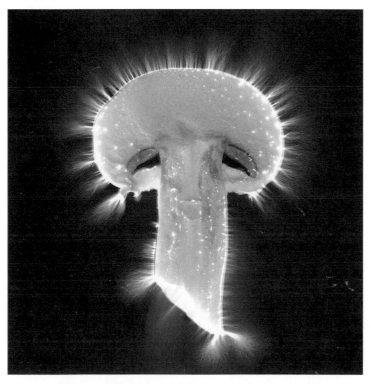

Raw Organic Mushroom *(Kirlian Image)*

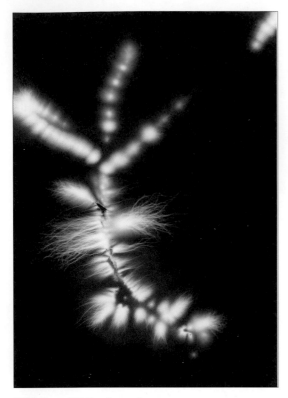

Wild Grass (*Kirlian Image*)

Wild Food

The ancient Greek poet, Hesiod, wrote about his ancestors, "the uncultivated fields afforded them their fruits, and supplied their bountiful and unenvied repast."

Just a few thousand years ago, 100% of the human population was eating 100% wild food! Agriculture did not exist.

Picking wild berries, fruits, and vegetables (*such as dandelion*) makes for a wonderful hobby. It reconnects us with nature in a simple and enjoyable way.

Wild food contains more minerals than organic food. If one is not able to pick wild fruits and vegetables for at least 25% of the diet, it is recommended to include a 100% raw organic green superfood powder in the diet and fresh juices to supply a full spectrum of minerals and nutrients.

Fresh Juices

Fresh juices filled with chlorophyll from green-leafy foods (*such as celery, parsley, spinach, kale, broccoli, etc.*) and fruits (*such as apples or pears to sweeten*) are a wonderful way to begin and maintain a beautiful body for a lifetime.

The habit of drinking fresh vegetable juices daily is probably the fastest way to transform your body and succeed with The Beauty Diet®. Remember that, to utilize the nutrients in food, that food must first be turned into a liquid. Juicing quickens the digestive process and delivers nutrients more quickly to your bloodstream.

To educate yourself on juices, I invite you to read some books on the subject. One of the best books on juicing is Steve Meyerowitz's *Power Juices Super Drinks*.

Proper Chewing

Complete nutrition and perfect digestion begin in the mouth with excellent chewing. Remember to chew your food well and convert it to a liquid before swallowing. One saying goes, "Drink your food, chew your juice." Another says, "Chew your food well, for the stomach has no teeth." Constipation, which is an epidemic in society, begins when one fails to chew food excellently.

Proper Food Combining

With reference to food combinations, it is always best to eat simply. Generally, sweet fruits should be eaten alone. Green-leafy vegetables and fats/oils tend to go well together. We seem to instinctively enjoy avocado with a salad or olive oil with a salad.

If any cooked food is eaten, it should be one type of cooked food eaten with a salad. For example, a sandwich with bread, meat, and cheese is a classic miscombination. Having just the bread with a sandwich containing avocado, sprouts, tomato, cucumber, and lettuce is a much better combination. Another example is to have just rice with a salad, instead of having both rice and fish for dinner. Just this simple advice can make a world of difference in one's digestion and overall health.

If you are totally new to the concept of food combining, I recommend that you read *Food Combining And Digestion* by Steve Meyerowitz, and *Food Combining Made Easy* by Dr. Herbert Shelton.

Variety

Each plant mines a different spectrum of minerals and provides a different type of nutrition. Eat a wide variety of different foods. Primates in nature eat approximately 115 different types of raw-plant-foods each year and 25 different types of raw-plant-foods each week. These are great target numbers for us to achieve as well.

Every food should be eaten in a rotation, everything in an ebb-and-flow pattern. Always keep in mind the concepts of rotation *(not too much of any one food)*, eating a wide variety of food, and easing into things slowly *(the body rejects sudden changes)*. We benefit by eating with the seasons and by nourishing ourselves with the food nature provides in each season.

Remember, if you find that a food I recommend does not agree with you, choose another that does.

Restoring Food Instincts

In today's world, some people consider the insatiable desire for pizza pie to be the ultimate experience of "instinct"!

Our instinct or intuition is located in our tummy area — sometimes called our "gut." That is why we have the sayings, "My gut instinct is telling me this," or "My gut feeling is telling me that."

Most people are not in touch with their instinct or intuition because their tummies *(guts)* are filled with so much "insulation" and excess waste.

My goal is simply to provide tools *(certainly not rules)* to help guide you from point A to point B on your dietary journey. Point A being a place of uncertainty as to what the body actually desires and when, and point B being the natural state. Once you reach point B, you will have cleansed yourself to a significant degree, and your food instincts, or intuition, will be aligned so that you may guide yourself more accurately into the future. You will have regained contact with your raw instincts, the same instincts that all the creatures possess in the wilds of nature.

Our inner computer is incredibly accurate if we avoid gumming up our inner circuitry with poor foods.

As you progress to a healthier state, you will find that you should be careful when things do not feel right. When you are indecisive about what to eat, eat nothing. If your intuition tells you to avoid something, avoid it.

Intestinal Cleansing

The benefits of The Beauty Diet® increase as one eliminates toxic foods from the diet and nurtures a healthy digestive system that will properly assimilate nutrients.

While it has been popular to undergo face lifts, tummy tucks, botox, and "pill popping" to achieve lasting youth, these only address symptoms, instead of real causes.

The primary cause of problem skin, excess fat, quickened aging, and poor muscle quality is toxemia — an accumulation of toxic substances in the tissues and intestines. Toxemia may have been fostered by stress, a poor diet, a lack of exercise, and/or other factors.

Toxemia is relieved by removing physical congestion from the small intestines through herbal cleansing.

A challenge with going on a raw-food diet without cleansing is that when an individual begins to move into a raw-food regime, s/he begins to cleanse at the microscopic cellular level, but not sufficiently at the macroscopic level *(intestinal tract)*.

I recommend that at the six month point of following the guidelines in this book (*eating raw-plant-food, drinking water, including super-foods in the diet*), it is time to do an EJUVA intestinal cleanse program. This is a one-month herbal program that you adopt into your daily routine. Complete instructions are included with each kit. This program assists your body in clearing away macroscopic accumulated debris in the intestines. The results are remarkable and self-evident. The EJUVA system is 100% raw and organic.

Cleansing with an herbal system, such as EJUVA, will help clear away not only physical blockages, but emotional issues as well. When one feels physically stronger and more nour-ished, it is easier to heal emotional issues.

When one completes a cleanse, energy flows cleanly through the body. The charis-matic qualities of bliss, joy, and happiness arise more easily. You will feel a change in your thoughts, emotions, judgements and motivations. One's focus and concentration are naturally drawn to higher things. You will eventually discover that there is no limit to how healthy and happy we can be. This process allows you to go beyond perfect health and totally transform your appearance if you are committed.

Parasite Cleansing

Often a parasitic infection is at the bottom of a particularly long-standing illness or weakness.

Parasites are able to live in our digestive systems when the bowels are not moving fre-quently enough. In the northern hemisphere the primary source of parasites comes from consuming meat and fish — especially when eaten raw.

Carnivores have a short digestive tract. In a carnivore's digestive tract, the parasite lar-vae in meat and fish are not able to hatch as easily, because the food moves out in 3 to 8 hours. The long, plant-friendly digestive tract of humans, and the 17 to 24 hours (*or 2 to 3 days if we are unhealthy*) it takes to move

food through, allows time for parasite larvae to hatch.

After three to six months on this beauty program, it is important that everyone do a parasite cleanse. A parasite cleanse may con-sist of a combination of various anti-parasite herbs taken daily. These herbs may primarily include: raw garlic, aged garlic extracts as well as whole powdered wormwood, cloves, and black walnut hull.

Enzymes

Enzymes are protein-based molecules that act as biological catalysts. On a physical level they help transform one molecule into anoth-er, and even help transform one element into another. On a spiritual level, enzymes are the symbol of transformation. They can help move one out of stagnation. In fact, enzymes should be thought of as the necessary element in moving stagnation out of the body — whether that is in the form of excess weight, toxins, or even repetitive negative thoughts.

Only raw-foods and enzyme supplements contain enzymes. All enzymes are destroyed by the cooking process, causing food to liter-ally "stick to our ribs."

Digestive enzymes are an excellent transi-tion tool to have in the beauty cabinet. This is because they allow for complete digestion. As Viktoras Kulvinskas, author of *Survival Into The 21st Century*, states, "What you don't digest, you wear on your skin."

Myself in conjunction with Sunfood Nutrition (www.sunfood.com) have devel-oped a product called *Beauty Enzymes*™, based on the leading-edge research of the pio-neers in the field. *Beauty Enzymes*™ are the most powerful combination of digestive and metabolic enzymes ever developed. This enzyme blend should be taken with any cooked food (*digestive*) and between meals when possible (*metabolic*). I recommend mov-ing toward an 80%-100% raw-food approach over time and when appropriate. Digestive enzyme supplements are still beneficial even when eating 100% raw-foods.

The Probiotic Revolution

Our intestines must be inhabited by friendly bacteria *(probiotics and soil organisms)* to help us digest food and produce nutrients, such as all B vitamins and vitamin K. They crowd out unfriendly bacteria and create the sound basis for good nutrition.

A healthy adult can have more than 400 species of good bacteria in the digestive tract. In total, they may weigh more than 2.5 kilograms *(5 pounds)* and exceed the number of cells in the body by 10 times. In essence, in a healthy body, the total number of bacteria in the digestive tract greatly exceeds all the cells in the body.

Digestion 101

In the normal progression of the life cycle, the human baby would first be fed mother's milk, thus the entire intestinal tract would be saturated with mother's probiotics *(such as Bifidus infantis)*. The next step for the baby would be the beginning of crawling, playing in the dirt, and putting her/his hands in the mouth. At that stage, in a natural environment, friendly soil-based organisms would colonize the intestines. With both the probiotics and friendly soil-based organisms in place, the stage is set for perfect food digestion and a strong immune system.

If we were fed formula instead of mother's milk, if we grew up in cities without the connection with our food and the soil, if we took antibiotics *(antibiotics kill both friendly and unfriendly bacteria)*, and if we ate foods high in sugar *(contributes to fungus/candida)*, then we can be assured that we will greatly benefit from taking in probiotic bacteria in a supplemental form.

Once we understand this logic, it is easy to see why digestive disruption is typically caused by low quantities of good bacteria, the lingering effects of antibiotics, refined sugar, alcohol, haphazard food combining *(always keep meals simple)*, carbonated beverages, chemical food additives, and drugs.

— The Perfect — Intestinal Environment

Have you ever seen rich, vibrant soil that smells incredible? The flora in the intestines should resemble the microbes found in rich black soil — rich and filled with life. As your intestines build up to — and match — that kind of microbe richness, your digestion will astound you.

The human body is an amazing farmer of good intestinal bacteria *(flora)*. You are a farmer. You farm your intestinal flora. A bad attitude can create storms that can wipe out your harvest. A poor diet can create floods that can wipe out your best farmland. Antibiotics are pesticides that eventually destroy your delicate soil. Anger acidifies your soil. A lack of health disciplines allows weeds to invade your farm. Patience, consistency, and persistence bring forth an amazing harvest. Sometimes, simply not eating for a day or two *(fasting)* allows the internal balance to restore itself.

The soil and intestines should contain many of the same organisms. A lack of soil organisms in the intestines leads to a disconnection between what is going on in the intestines and what is going on in the soil. This is the physical reason why many people feel or behave as if they have become "disconnected" from the planet.

That picture of rich soil is what we can picture in our minds when we are thinking about maintaining excellent digestion. Picture perfect health — richness, vibrancy, lots of healthy microbes.

— Probiotics —

Probiotics are extremely effective at combating parasites, fungus, mold, and yeast in the body and the digestive tract.

Different probiotics have different specific effects. The probiotic *L. salivarius* seems to be particularly powerful in cleansing the colon. *L. salivarius* seems to be able to eat away harmful mucus accumulations in the intestines more effectively than any other type of good bacteria. Other probiotics, such as *Bifidus infantis, B. bifidum,* and *B. longum* are effective in normalizing the intestinal pH while driving out fungus and mold.

— Soil Organisms —

Soil microbes come with our fruits, vegetables, and herbs when they are picked fresh and eaten unwashed — the way we have always eaten from the beginning of time. This is the way garden eating should be done.

Usually, any fresh foods purchased from a store should be washed with pure water and diluted *(0.5%)*, food-grade hydrogen peroxide *(not the brown bottles)*. This is due to the fact that by the time the food has traveled to the food store, it has probably been affected by mold or fungus lingering in trucks and/or refrigerators.

Soil organisms are resistant to stomach acids and are able to implant no matter how much bad bacteria is present in the digestive tract. These organisms are stable enough to survive in an alkaline colon.

Soil organisms and probiotics help repair and restore the villi of the small intestine, which are responsible for absorbing nutrients. These organisms contain vitamin A, vitamin B12, anti-inflammatory gamma-linolenic acid *(GLA)* and super oxide dismutase *(SOD — an incredibly powerful antioxidant).*

Soil organisms and probiotics boost the immune system by producing immune weapons such as anti-viral alpha-interferon, iron-delivering lactoferrin, T-cells, and antibodies.

— Probiotics and Soil Organisms —

Probiotics and soil organisms are each effective in:

1. Preventing growth of harmful bacteria, yeast, fungi, etc.

2. Maintaining the chemical and hormonal balance within the body.

3. Producing and regulating vitamins *(especially B vitamins, including vitamin B12).*

4. Assisting the digestive system.

5. Aiding the proper function of the immune system and correcting nutritional deficiencies.

6. Decreasing body odor. This is because probiotic bacteria eat away and digest putrefaction. A friend of mine feeds probiotics to her two dogs and as a result her dogs have no body or breath odor.

—Simplicity —

To simplify everything, I promote a product called *Sun Is Shining Superfood*, which was developed in order to meet several needs all at once. *Sun Is Shining Superfood* contains superfoods, enzymes, and probiotics, allowing one to obtain all these amazing elements in one source.

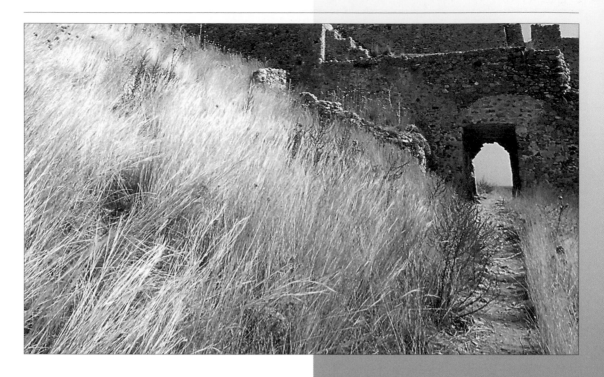

DETOXIFICATION & TRANSFORMATION

Raw-plant-foods, medicinal herbs, laughter, bliss, joy, and unconditional love all exist in the same frequency. Tuning into this frequency raises the overall vibration of your energy field, causing anything that is vibrating at a lower frequency, such as fear, pain, doubt, cancer, ugliness, depression, toxins, and so on, to eventually percolate out and be ejected from the body. This process is known as "detoxification."

Detoxification transforms us, yet also challenges us. As you embark and continue into this process, remember that you do not need to focus on perfection, just progress. Old habits die hard, but they do die. Some shifts will happen immediately, while others will take time. The path may be relatively easy or it may be challenging.

Inner cleansing, detoxification, and body awareness are all by-products of embarking on a raw-food program. The results provide the instructions and inspire one to proceed further and further.

The transformative process that begins by eating raw-plant-foods allows you to

"Feed him with apricots and dewberries,

With purple grapes, green figs and mulberries."

— *Shakespeare*
(These are the words of Titania admonishing her fairies when she wished to purge Bottom of his "mortal grossness" in *A Midsummer Night's Dream*)

rebuild yourself at a deep level. It allows you to reshape yourself into a more perfect work of art. It endows you with a new-found ability to resculpt your character, physique, and future. It inspires you to fully invest your time into the process of recreating yourself as a masterpiece.

The Flight of Daedalus

We all know the mythical story of the "Flight of Icarus." Remember? Icarus was caught in the labyrinth on the island of Crete. His father, Daedalus, a master engineer, created wings for his son so that he could fly back with him and escape. His father told him "fly the middle way. Do not fly too high, or the Sun will melt the wax on your wings, and you'll fall from the sky. Do not fly too low, or the tides of the sea will catch you." The two donned the wings and flew off the island together. Icarus, however, became ecstatic in flight and flew too high. The wax on the wings melted, and he plummeted into the sea.

This story is often called the "Flight of Icarus," yet from now on you may remember it as the "Flight of Daedalus," because it was Daedalus who succeeded! Daedalus was brave, he took action. But he was also smart, unlike Icarus who did not listen. The lesson here is to take a chance, to fly, and also to listen closely and educate yourself. Raw-foods is powerful information, and by adopting this program you will fly — make sure you listen and stay educated.

To be able to handle the metabolic change that occurs when shifting to a raw-food-based diet, you need to move at your own pace and begin where you are. Consistently move that pace up as you are able.

Handle yourself like a wise manager does when bringing a promising prize fighter along — he makes sure that his prize fighter does not face anyone in his early bouts who could knock him out. Push yourself along at a pace that your confidence and ability can handle.

Minor victories lead to major victories. Small commitments lead to large commitments. An object in motion tends to stay in motion, whether it is a train, a car, an emotion, a habit, or a belief. One step leads to another. Each triumph brings you one step

closer to realizing the goal of eternal youth and beauty.

All changes should be adopted with common sense. Too sudden of a shift can "shock" the body. Everything comes as it should, in its own time. The way to create lasting change is to step outside of your comfort zone, but not into your shock zone.

A word to the wise:
Habit does advise
That a sudden shift
May be too swift.

A shift's gift
May stir and uplift
Things of the past,
Best released slow
Instead of fast.

When you continue to strive
Slow changes arrive,
Persistency is like a gauge,
Step-by-step, page-by-page,
Consistency is nature's wage
That unlocks any cage.

If you want to realize greater health gains, invest your time and efforts in detoxification efforts and personal-development projects that develop over a long period of time. The long-range projects pay off so much more because the universe rewards the virtues of discipline and perseverance.

Symptoms of Detoxification

"If you're going through hell, keep going."
— *Winston Churchill*

Headaches, body aches, skin challenges, excess mucus, PMS, body odor, halitosis, bowel irregularities, feelings of discomfort, emotional fluctuations, lack of interest in sex, deep doubts, and soul searching are all symptoms of detoxification that may occur in cycles. These are symptoms of low energy phenomenon being flushed out by higher energy foods and emotions.

Have you ever stepped into a calm pond or lake in the early morning hours? Once you step in, the mud at the bottom is churned up. Detoxification is like this. Eating healthy, lighter foods churns up the old sludge, including past old emotional residue and buried hurt. Emotional cleansing is part of the transformation process.

If you are experiencing strong detoxification symptoms — especially through the skin — visit a colon hydrotherapist. Colonics can help channel and remove the toxicity and emotions through the bowels instead of the skin.

How To Slow Down or Speed Up Detoxification Symptoms

Catabolic practices tend to speed up or accelerate detoxification symptoms (*this means that a catabolic practice will move toxins through and out of the body faster*). "Catabolic" means "to break down."

Catabolic Practices Include...

- Fasting
- Eating sweet fruit
- Drinking green juices
- Drinking only water
- Aerobic exercise
- Herbal cleansing
- Hot springs bathing
- Sweatlodge/Sauna
- Colon hydrotherapy
- Massage
- Orgasm
- Skin brushing
- Taking enzymes and probiotic supplements
- Taking MSM (*methyl-sulfonyl-methane*) as a supplement

Anabolic practices tend to slow down detoxification (*this means that an anabolic practice will suppress the release of toxins from the body*). "Anabolic" means "to build up."

Anabolic Practices Include...

- Eating fatty foods (*avocados, nuts, olives, seeds, coconuts, durian*)
- Eating fibrous green-leafy vegetable salads
- Using sea salt
- Anaerobic exercise, such as heavy weight lifting
- Eating cooked starches like bread, pasta, rice, baked potato, etc.
- Eating any kind of dairy product
- Eating any type of meat, including fish

Neither catabolic nor anabolic practices are more important than each other. They are both valuable and useful at the correct time.

A Lesson in Detachment

Rid your home and workspace of anything that you have not used or touched in the last year.

Have you ever walked into someone's home and seen stuff everywhere? Stuff on the counters, stuff on the walls, stuff in the closet, stuff on the floor? Heaven help you if you should open the refrigerator! Stuff! Guess what is inside the person who lives amongst all this? Lots of stuff!

What we see around us is only a reflection of what is inside of us. If we see clutter around us, the tendency is for clutter to be present within us.

There is a special healing force in detachment, in letting go. In my journeys I have discovered that success is not about what you get, it is about what you let go of. Letting go of objects around us allows us to let go of "stuff" within us — it helps with the detoxification process.

Detoxification Is Personal

Self-healing through alternative healthcare and alternative dermatology is a very personal and awakening study. Alternative healthcare sciences tend to view people as whole individuals in an environment with a history, rather than as a group of labeled symptoms and diagnoses.

Use your intuition/instincts to aid your choice of naturopaths, physicians, or healers. If you feel that more esoteric healing regimes are appropriate, such as prayer, psychics, faith, or another alternative method, then by all means act upon that feeling. This is where you may have your greatest breakthroughs.

Allow your feelings to aid you in the choice of doctors and healing techniques. Naturopathic healing techniques are powerful. Even faith and psychic healing may have its role in your life. There is an extraordinary intelligence among us. The greatest benefit of natural and spiritual healing regimes is the adventuresome, optimistic frame of mind that arises from their use.

Weight Loss

Enlightenment is just that — making yourself lighter.

Permanent weight loss comes through an inner transformation. This usually arises from an epiphany, a moment of clarity, a clear decision. When the decision has been made and a new path in life is chosen, the weight is already lost.

The two biggest elements to limit and eliminate in the diet in order to lose weight are: starchy carbohydrates such as baked potatoes, rice, beer, bread, pasta, corn chips, potato chips, etc., and cooked fats such as high-fat meat and pasteurized dairy foods.

Overeating habits and weight gain are related to eating demineralized foods. The richer a food is in minerals, the more difficult it becomes to overeat it. When food is eaten raw, it gives a stronger signal to stop eating.

This is called the "aliesthetic taste change." This taste change is stronger in more mineralized foods and is especially strong in wild foods. It is virtually impossible to overeat wild foods. Wild foods are always higher in minerals than domesticated foods. Domesticated plants, especially those that are commercially grown, tend to be high in sugar/starch and low in minerals. These include grains (*bread, pasta, rice-cakes, beer*), potatoes (*baked, potato chips*), corn (*corn chips, corn syrup products*), carrots, and seedless fruits. The consumption of demineralized food often leads to addictions. I remember being addicted to corn chips while in college, which actually caused a subtle inflammation in my skin.

Hypothyroidism (*an underactive thyroid gland*) has been the target of much of the blame for excessive weight gain. This can be true, though it is not always the case. If indeed thyroid challenges are at the cause of excessive weight, the best course of action is to feed the thyroid with coconut oil (*as well as other coconut products*), kelp, brazil nuts (*3 to 4 each day*), fruits rich in vitamin C (*oranges, peppers*), and foods high in B vitamins and enzymes (*raw sauerkraut*).

How To Cut Cellulite Fast

Drink only fresh grapefruit juice or simply eat only grapefruits for three days. Grapefruits contain the wonderful anti-inflammatory and skin-cleansing enzyme bromelain. Grapefruits are the mildest citrus fruit in acid-content, yet they retain the strong antiseptic, mucus-dissolving properties found in all citrus fruits. They are also mild in sugar content, making them gentle on the pancreas as well as blood-sugar levels.

Another strategy is to eat frugally (*lightly*) and take two Beauty Enzymes™ with every meal and two between meals to build up the cleansing protease and lipase enzyme levels in the tissues helping to break down cellulite and excess fat. Avoid taking enzymes on an empty stomach if you have a history of ulcers.

You Can Transform

The miraculous thing about us is that we are dynamic beings. We rebuild ourselves constantly. General wisdom holds that 98% of the atoms in our bodies are replaced in two years. Studies have shown that 100% of our atomic structure is replaced within seven years!

Now comes the startling truth: You can change your bone structure; you can greatly alter your appearance; you can change the mold of your flesh to suit your ideals. We all become the image we hold of ourselves within our own minds. In spite of all the doubters and disbelievers, this is the truth I have come to know based on my own experiences with raw-food and my own physical transformation.

My promise to you is that excellent organic, highly-mineralized, raw-food choices practiced consistently will transform you in two years by replacing your atomic structure with the correct building materials. In seven years you will be entirely transformed into a new person.

All knowledge and learning amount to little when compared to the need to purify and rejuvenate the body at all levels — physical, mental, emotional, and spiritual — because a renewed body is capable of accessing the deepest wisdom. Everyone who chooses to purify themselves receives rewards beyond their imagination — if they are willing to progress intelligently and pass the tests. It is through this process of self-purification that we become beings of pure essential beauty.

At present, most of us are completely unaware of what true beauty and charisma can truly do. With enough charisma and purity, there is no limitation. Enough charisma creates opportunities at every turn. It generates unique and magical events each day.

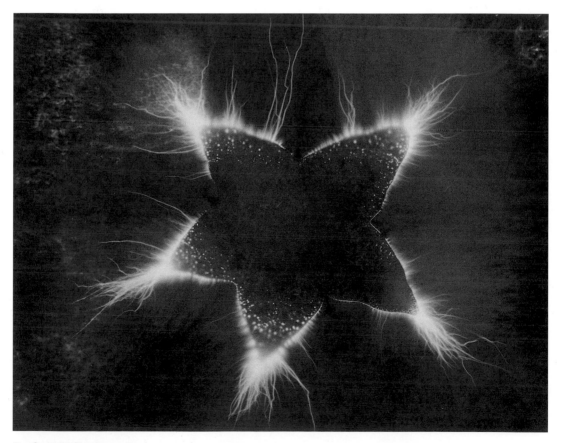

Starfruit *(Kirlian Image)*

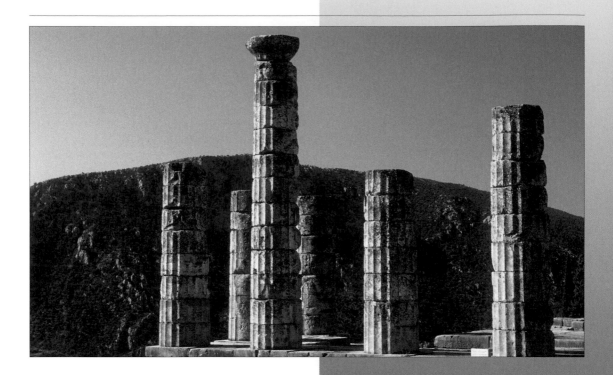

ALCHEMICAL BEAUTY SECRETS

The Beauty Minerals

*B*eauty depends on mineralization. People living where minerals are rich in the food tend to also be the most beautiful. Consider the beauty of the Nordics living beneath the glaciers, the Africans from volcanically-rich areas, and the Pacific Islanders and Native Americans on their indigenous diets.

Minerals, in an assimilable form, are required for rejuvenation and beauty. If minerals come through to us in the form of plants, then the body can assimilate them and utilize them immediately. Daily ingesting large quantities of colloidal minerals in liquid form can create trace mineral overdoses. Take those minerals and put them in your garden, then eat the plants.

Becoming more deeply mineralized is a step-by-step process. It involves slowly opening up your body to assimilate more minerals by eating more and more mineral-rich foods. It involves taking in more mineralized food over years of time. It involves taking in all the co-factors that naturally come with the minerals in their living state *(as they would be found in raw plants).* It involves moving to organic foods, organic superfoods, and beyond. In particular it involves saturating one's tissues with the beauty minerals silicon, sulfur, zinc, and iron.

The Theory of the Elements

Different elements *(otherwise called atoms or minerals)* are given different names and are usually represented by their first letter. When there are several elements with the same first letter, they are distinguished by adding another letter from the name of the element. For example, C = Carbon, Ca = Calcium, Cl = Chlorine, Cu = Copper *(derived from the French cuivre)*, S = Sulfur, Si = Silicon, N = Nitrogen, Na = Natrium *(Sodium)*.

Gold is represented by Au, from the Latin "aurum." Mercury is represented by Hg, from the name for mercury poisoning — hydrargyrism.

Some elements, like Potassium *(which is represented by the letter K)* are drawn from their more ancient names. Potassium is derived from the Latin word "Kalium" — which is derived from the Arabic "al Khali." This word has been brought into English as "alkali" — a strong base *(the opposite of a strong acid)*. This is where our word "alkaline" originates. *(Special note: potassium is chemically alkaline, though not an alkaline mineral in food)*.

Minerals differ from compounds and molecules. Compounds and molecules consist of combinations of minerals. For example, silica is a combination of silicon and oxygen — SO_2. Chemical water is a combination of hydrogen and oxygen — H_2O. Ammonia is a combination of nitrogen and hydrogen — NH_3.

Biological Transmutations

The late Nobel-prize nominee and French professor, C.L. Kervran *(member of the New York Academy of Sciences, Director of Conferences at Paris University)* revolutionized the field of biology and minerals through his research beginning in 1959 and ending with his death in 1983. His interest in the concept of biological transmutations *(alchemical changes created by living organisms)* began when he was a child. In his book, *Biological Transmutations*, he describes, "My parents kept some hens in a shed with free access to a yard. We lived in central Brittany, where my father was a civil servant. The district was one of schist and granite, devoid of limestone. Limestone was never given to the chickens, but every day they produced eggs with a calcareous shell. I never thought of asking where the calcium of the egg came

from *(nor the calcium in the bones of the birds)*. But I was intrigued by an observation I had made. When the laying hens were loose in the yard, they pecked incessantly at the flakes of mica which dotted the ground. *(Mica, together with quartz and feldspar, is a constituent of granite. They are all compounds of silica. That was all I knew at the time, when I was at primary school.)* I noticed this evident selection of mica by the hens when the sun was shining after a shower. Well washed by the rain, the hundreds of flakes visible in each square meter looked like miniature mirrors, and the pecking of the hens was easy to follow. No one could tell me why the birds pecked the mica and not the grains of sand. I watched my mother opening the gizzard after a fowl had been killed and saw small stones and sand inside, but never mica. Where had the mica gone? This made an impression on me, and like everything which remains a mystery, stayed in my subconscious mind. Being a child, I liked solid logical explanations — the reason why."

C.L. Kervran eventually discovered what was happening with the chickens. The enzymes in their digestive system were transmutating silicon into calcium.

Biological transmutation is the ability to transmutate one element into another alchemically *(i.e. organic silica into calcium, potassium into sodium, manganese into iron, etc.)*. C.L. Kervran simply uncovered biological transmutations — a phenomenon that had been there all along.

Life, we have found, is more than just chemistry and physics. In every field there always seems to be a new random factor, an insight, similar to what we find with the raw-food paradigm displacing present nutrition ideas. The idea that atomic minerals can be changed from one to another is generally termed alchemy. Alchemical transformations pertain neither to chemistry nor nuclear physics in their present understanding.

Present-day science has a prejudice against this idea. The idea that minerals remain atomically stable, unless there is radiation, is generally termed "Lavoisier's Law." Lavoisier's

Law states, "Nothing is lost, nothing is created, everything is transformed." In chemistry this may be true, but in biological chemistry it has been discovered that this is not true.

With due respect to the scientific prejudice that pervades academics, it is not my goal to convince anyone of biological transmutations. I am only interested in results. If something works, then an explanation is really just an intellectual exercise.

Biological transmutations are directly in line with the rapid advancement in all the sciences. One must resist all traditional scientific orthodoxy in light of what we know about the history of science. All science has always been changing based on new evidence. As long as what is reported can be demonstrated, then we must move forward with more precise theories. Only results matter, not theories.

For information on elemental transmutations, please refer to C. L. Kervran's landmark book, *Biological Transmutations (a compilation of his 5 books and over 5,000 pages of notes),* and also Wilfred Branfield's book, *Continuous Creation.*

Silicon

"The ability of silica to change into limestone has been recognized for ages, since in antiquity horsetail *(equisetum)* was used for recalcification. *(Horsetail is rich in silica.)* It was also used for curing tuberculosis because it speeds up calcification of the lung caverns, thus promoting quicker healing. In 1846, Pierre Jousset, one of the great masters of homeopathy, showed in a thesis the effect of silica on people stricken with tuberculosis."

— *Professor C.L. Kervran,*
Biological Transmutations

Knowledge of biological transmutations gives us an advantage. Within this phenomenon we find one of the world's greatest beauty secrets — that the mineral silicon possesses many hidden properties, one of which is its ability to be transformed into calcium.

Silicon is a conscious mineral. It seems to possess a form of intelligence. This is why all our computers are coming from "Silicon Valley" and are based on silicon technology. This is also why crystals and crystal healing are so popular *(crystals are made of silicon)*. It is also why silicon possesses such incredible healing and beautifying properties. Many believe that ingesting foods high in this mineral has a tendency to expand awareness and manifest a more perfect physical appearance.

— What Silicon Does in the Body —

Silicon is present in blood vessels, bones, cartilage, connective tissue, hair, ligaments, lungs, lymph nodes, muscles, nails, skin, teeth, tendons, and trachea.

Silicon, being an incredible insulator, keeps the blood warm and helps to direct the flow of electricity imparted through the electrolyte salts in the blood. It helps to maintain the elasticity of arterial cell walls.

In bones, silicon is found in areas of active growth. Growing and healing bones may contain high levels of silicon at the calcification site *(for reasons we have noted above, namely, that silicon is transformed into calcium)*. Silicon-rich foods and herbs *(such as horsetail, nettles, oat straw, and hemp leaf)* have been shown to increase bone-mineral density.

A silicon-rich diet — especially in children — leads to beautiful teeth and jaw formation. Silicon helps prevent cavities. Silicon also helps prevent bleeding gums and gum atrophy that allow the teeth to loosen, which could ultimately lead to tooth loss. My experience has been that large quantities of foods rich in silicon, along with daily raw-food nutrition and proper dental hygiene can even reverse the formation of cavities.

Silicon is a yoga mineral. Healthy muscle tissues contain at least 2% silicon, allowing for flexibility and elasticity.

Connective tissue consists of collagen, elastin, and polysaccharide sugars. All these important molecules harbor large quantities of silicon. These are the bonding elements that hold us together. They maintain the elastic quality of the skin, the tendons, and even of the eyes. The ability of connective tissue to retain moisture is obviously of major importance in the prevention of premature aging. This tissue "juiciness" is dependent upon raw-food nutrition, hydration, and the presence of silicon.

The highest concentration of silicon is found in the hair and nails. A 1993 study found the oral and external application of silicon improves the condition of aging skin, hair, and nails in women. Silicon increased the thickness and strength of the skin, improved wrinkles, and gave hair and nails a healthier appearance.

Generally, one is more youthful when there is more silicon in relationship to calcium present in the body. The ratio of silicon to calcium is a biological marker of youth. At birth, the body has a large supply of the youth mineral silicon, and low calcium. With age, the ratio reverses. Studies done on the human aorta show that by age ten, due to the present-day demineralized diet, much silicon is already lost, and it declines even more with age.

Next to oxygen, silicon is the most abundant element on earth. It appears as oxide silica in sand and quartz, and as silicates in minerals such as granite. Paradoxically, it only appears in large concentrations in certain foods.

— Silicon-Rich Foods —

- Young bamboo (bamboo shoots)
- Horsetail
- Hemp leaves
- Nettles
- Oatstraw
- Mature blades of grass (found often in superfood powders)
- Alfalfa
- Radish
- Nopal cactus
- Romaine lettuce
- Marjoram
- New Zealand spinach
- Burdock root
- Cucumbers (found in the fruit's skin)
- Bell peppers (found in the fruit's skin)
- Tomatoes (found in the fruit's skin)
- Young tender green plants in springtime
- Oats (steel-cut oatmeal is best)
- Sun Is Shining Superfood

Best Silicon Supplements
(best taken with whole-food vitamin C)

- Sunfood Nutrition's Ormus Gold *(this "ten-years-in-development" product includes silica)*

- Orgono Living Silica *(a liquid miracle)*

- Flora's Premium Vegetal Silica contains a water soluble, aqueous extract of the herb horsetail. This supplement is formulated using the method developed by Professor C. L. Kervran.

Signs of a Silicon Deficiency Include

- Poor skin quality
- Brittle nails and hair
- Dental cavities
- Weak bones
- Weak tendons and ligaments
- Atherosclerosis *(weak and porous arteries leading to cardiovascular disease)*
- Lung disorders *(emphysema)*

Sulfur

"In 1844 Vogel experimented with watercress seeds placed under a large bell jar. Keeping the air 'analyzed,' he added a nutritive solution containing no sulfur whatsoever. After their germination he analyzed the young plants, finding that they contained more sulfur than the seed from which they stemmed. This phenomenon remained obscure to Vogel, who concluded that either sulfur is not a simple body or there was an unknown source of sulfur."

— *Professor C.L. Kervran, Biological Transmutations*

Experiments I have performed in nature have proven to me that plants in the mustard family *(broccoli, arugula, mustard, radish, etc.)* create sulfur. These plants can form sulfur compounds in heavy concentrations where no sulfur is present in the soil, and in desert conditions where sulfur from rainfall is minimal.

Professor C.L. Kervran concluded that sulfur can actually be formed from a "fritting" of two oxygen atoms into an atom of sulfur. Sulfur, in fact, still retains oxygenating properties. Sulfur compounds are spicy. They tend to cleanse our tissues in a way that they feel "oxygenated." Oxygen and sulfur are more closely related than most scholars currently understand. This is just one of the mysterious properties of sulfur.

Strange odors in nature, especially near hot springs, are produced by sulfur compounds.

Of all the major minerals, sulfur is one of the least discussed, yet one of the most important.

— What Sulfur Does in the Body —

Sulfur is the foundational mineral of all beauty. It produces a flame-like tint in the skin. It creates a subtle lustre as delicate as the halo around the full moon on a clear desert evening. It carries with it a certain elegance and aristocracy. Sulfur-residue foods make the complexion radiant.

In nature, sulfur is found in MSM *(methyl-sulfonyl-methane)*, a sulfur compound found in the oceans, rain water, and all living things. It is also found in the following amino acids: methionine, taurine, cysteine, and cystine. The latter three amino acids can be made by the body from methionine, MSM, and/or sulfur-rich foods. Sulfurous amino acids protect us against the effects of radiation and heavy metals. Methionine helps draw heavy metals out of the body. Methionine is found in high concentrations in raw pumpkin seeds. Cystine and cysteine are found in hemp seeds. They are closely related and are nearly identical. Cystine is present in hair, keratin, and insulin. Cystine makes up about 14% of the skin and hair. Cysteine is present in the skin, making it more flexible, and in the collagen, helping to protect these tissues from damage. Scar tissue results without adequate cysteine.

Sulfur plays a major role in the bile fluid, brain, connective tissue *(collagen)*, hair, liver, nails, pancreas, and skin. Sulfur is generally considered to be the 8th or 9th most abundant mineral in the body. It is stored in every cell in the body and is especially highly concentrated in the joints, hair, skin, and nails. Adequate sulfur intake has a great deal to do with a beautiful complexion, mineralized hair, and glowing skin.

— Collagen and Elasticity —

Sulfur is an essential component of all connective tissue. Connective tissue supports and connects all the internal organs. Collagen is the protein found in the connective tissue, and also in the bones and teeth. Sulfur-rich collagen is the most common protein in the body. Collagen retains fluid and provides elasticity and flexibility to the tissues.

Sulfur compounds, such as glucosamine, give cartilage its strength, structure, and resilience. Glucosamine builds bone, ligaments, tendons, skin, eyes, and nails. Glucosamine is found in joint fluids.

Sulfur is found in keratin, a fibrous protein that makes up 98% of the nails. Sulfur in the form of keratin is also found in the skin, hair, nails, and in tooth enamel. Sulfur simultaneously gives these tissues greater strength and shape, as well as greater elasticity and flexibility.

— Hair, Nails, and Skin —

Essentially, through its ability to continuously build and rebuild perfect collagen and keratin, sulfur is able to make our hair, nails, and skin shine with radiance. Sulfur truly is the most beautifying of all food nutrients, and the best cosmetic in the world.

The curliness of one's hair depends on increasing the sulfur-to-sulfur bonds of the amino acid cystine. My hair is naturally curly, and my experience has demonstrated that from following the principles of The Beauty Diet® my hair has become more curly and shiny.

I have seen even the worst cases of acne clear up quickly *(sometimes in weeks)*, by switching to a raw-plant-food-based diet, taking in superfoods *(Pure Synergy or Sun Is Shining Superfood)*, including MSM in the diet, topically using small amounts of DMSO *(a very potent liquid form of MSM)*, adding camu camu berry as a vitamin C source, employing enzyme and probiotic supplementation, by topically using moderate quantities of MSM cream, and by properly opening and draining the lymph channels of the throat nick and clavicle via massage and/or magnetic stimulation. Even difficult internal and external scar tissue and burns can be broken down and repaired by following this protocol.

In general, bathing in hot springs water containing sulfur greatly enhances skin beauty. At the hot spring retreats we conduct, we often add to the experience by alternating hot with cold-water plunges into baths containing chaparral leaf tea to accelerate skin transformation and inner cleansing.

— Cell Permeability & Detoxification —

Sulfur regulates the sodium/potassium electrolyte balance in and out of the cell. This makes the cell more permeable and better able to drive nutrients into, and waste out of, the cell.

Sulfur helps relieve pain and inflammation by allowing waste products to be flushed out of the cell. Every time the body removes toxins from the cell, it also removes a sulfur compound that neutralizes the toxin. Therefore, sulfur is a vital mineral in the detoxification process.

— Blood Sugar —

Stable blood sugar is a major component of beauty because excess sugar damages collagen and excess sugar causes mood swings, leading to irritable behavior.

Sulfur is a component of insulin, which is the hormone that allows the uptake of glucose within cells for energy. Sulfur functions along with thiamine and biotin in a normal sugar metabolism. Hypoglycemia *(low blood sugar)* and diabetes are associated with a deficiency of sulfur at some level.

— Tissue Repair —

Sulfur provides elasticity, movement, healing, and repair within the tissues. Sulfur reduces lactic acid build up, and has the ability to reduce and possibly eliminate muscle, leg, and back cramps. Adequate sulfur levels in the diet can increase the speed of recovery in athletes by 75% as reported by Dr. Jacob *(the leading medical authority on MSM and co-author of The Miracle of MSM)*.

— Immune System —

Good bacterial flora *(probiotics)* use sulfur-residue foods to build various naturally-occurring body antibiotics to fight infections.

Sulfur also competes for binding receptor sites in the mucus membranes of the intestines, thus crowding out parasites *(giardia, trichomonads, roundworms, etc)*.

MSM
(Methyl-Sulfonyl-Methane)

MSM *(methyl-sulfonyl-methane)* is an organic form of sulfur that appears in all living organisms. One way it is formed is as a byproduct of algae growing in the oceans, and then is evaporated into clouds. As clouds precipitate, the MSM falls to the Earth and becomes food and nutrition for all life-forms on earth.

Because MSM is extremely volatile, and is either evaporated or destroyed by cooking, most people are extremely deficient in it. Even those who switch to raw-foods or even those who eat only raw-foods will benefit from additional MSM. Adequate volumes of sulfur are usually lacking in even a raw-food diet. This is because many foods are grown through irrigation and in greenhouses where they do not rely on the rain cycle, where much MSM originates. MSM is found in high concentrations only in plants that are watered by rain or sulfur-rich waters. Pine bark, pine needles, pine nuts, aloe vera, noni fruit, wild grasses, and fresh tobacco leaves *(not edible)* are some of the richest sources of MSM in nature.

MSM has been isolated and is now available in a supplemental crystal powder form. I had been eating a totally raw-food program for over four years when I began to include additional MSM in my diet. I started out small and gradually increased the dosage. I have experienced enough phenomenal results to radically alter my views on the importance of sulfur. The beautifying effects have been startling — no pimples, fast and thick hair growth on my face and scalp, no soreness in any muscles even after vigorous exercise, more elasticity for yoga, better brain function, and more.

MSM helps to alleviate pollen and food allergies. In fact, MSM neutralizes foreign proteins, such as pollen allergens, faster than anything else I have seen.

The sulfur concentration of arthritic tissue has been found to be 1/3 that of normal. MSM has been shown to help arthritic conditions by improving joint flexibility, reducing stiffness, reducing inflammation, reducing arthritic pain, and by breaking up scar tissue.

MSM is a potentiator. It makes all nutrients and supplements work better.

MSM greatly enhances the structural integrity of connective tissue and joint cartilage. It works synergistically with vitamin C to build new tissue.

MSM actually alters cross-linkages that create scars on the skin. MSM lotion applied topically is greatly beneficial in treating acne, dermatitis, eczema, psoriasis, rosacea, and scars.

Also, MSM lotion, because of its ability to neutralize foreign proteins, almost immediately neutralizes mosquito and insect bites. Test and be convinced.

— Recommended MSM Intake —

MSM appears to be completely safe, even in large doses. There are no known toxic effects from MSM.

Experience with MSM has shown that it works best when taken in small quantities initially *(1/4 to 1/2 tablespoon twice per day)* and then it should be built up to one, two, and even three tablespoons taken twice each day.

As with anything, shift slowly and then gradually, as your body opens to it, increase.

MSM has a natural affinity for water (*this is why it is lost when food has its water removed by heating*). Therefore, MSM is best taken by mixing it with your morning and afternoon glass of water.

— Sulfur-Residue Foods —

Adequate sulfur levels are maintained by including MSM and sulfur-residue foods regularly in one's diet, and sometimes, when instinct dictates, to include large doses. Sulfur-residue foods are commonly recognized by either their high protein content or their characteristic spicy, heating effect, evident in garlic, onion, mustard, horseradish, etc. The following is a list of sulfur-residue foods:

- Arugula
- Blue-green algae
  (*E3 Live Fresh algae or freeze/spray dried*)
- Bee pollen
  (*the most complete food found in nature*)
- Cabbage (*spicy*)
- Durian
- Hot chiles/peppers
- Broccoli
- Brussel sprouts
- Garlic
- Hemp seeds
- Horseradish
- Kale
- Maca
  (*superfood powder*)
- Mustard leaves
- Mustard, radish flowers
  (*very powerful sulfur source*)
- Many wild and domesticated cruciferous vegetables
  (*including broccoli, cauliflower, and kale*)

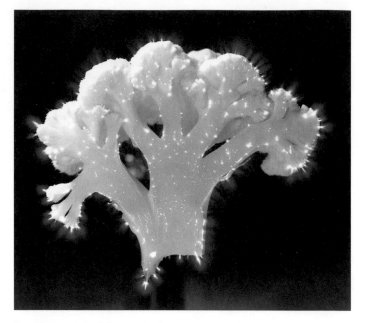

Raw Organic Cauliflower (*Kirlian Image*)

- Nasturtium
- Noni
- Onions
- Pumpkin seeds
- Radishes
  (*black, red, and daikon*)
- Spirulina
- Watercress

— How To Eat Sulfur-Residue Foods —

Sulfur-residue foods seem to be most assimilable if eaten in a certain way. If sulfur-residue foods are not eaten properly and/or not assimilated properly, they will promote fermentation in the intestines, leading to indigestion and gas. An excess of sulfurous foods containing mustard oils (*garlic, onions, hot peppers*) can cause a mild antiseptic mucus cleansing that may increase to a heavy discharge of mucus from the lungs and sinuses.

Sulfur is involved in the formation of bile acids, which are important for fat digestion and absorption. In fact, sulfurous foods combine well with fatty foods (*avocado, nuts, oil, some seeds, etc.*). The spicy sulfurous elements are softened by fats. This means that if one eats arugula in large quantities, then one may eat avocado or nuts with it to soften the harsh edge. Another example would be to include onions or garlic with avocado in a salad. This combining of a fatty food with a spicy sulfurous food is intuitive *(most people do it instinctively)*.

Sulfur-rich foods generate a subtle heating reaction; therefore, if overeaten they will overheat the intestines and cause gas. This can be balanced by bringing in an appropriate quantity of a salty vegetable *(at least as much or more of a salty vegetable as of the sulfur-residue food itself)*. Salty vegetables that calm down a sulfur reaction in the intestines include celery, kale, spinach, and chard.

Unwashed seaweeds contain a large amount of potassium and a large amount of sodium *(sea salt)*. Eating foods like this *(that are both high in potassium and sodium)* tends to diminish the sulfur reserves of the body because sulfur modifies the sodium/potassium balance. Essentially this means that seaweeds go well with high-sulfur foods.

To really make an amazing salad, one should follow the guideline above and include both a fatty-food *(avocados, nuts, oil, some seeds, etc.)*, a salty vegetable *(celery, kale, spinach, chard)*, and a seaweed *(dulse, nori, kelp)* with sulfur-residue foods. This makes everything assimilate and balance nicely. Experiment with different combinations to determine what works best for you.

Recipes are great. And knowing the theory behind recipes is even better. A "beauty salad" might contain:

- Lettuce
- Cauliflower
- Celery
- Arugula
- Onions
- Radishes
- Olives
- Burdock root
- Dulse seaweed
- Olive oil
- Lemon juice

Signs of a Sulfur Deficiency Include

- Acne
- Arthritis
- Brittle hair
- Brittle nails
- Gastro-intestinal challenges
- Immune dysfunction
- Lingering muscular injuries
- Lung dysfunctions due to inflammation
- Memory loss
- Rashes
- Scar tissue
- Slow wound healing

Many times symptoms that are labeled as a "protein deficiency" are in reality symptoms of a sulfur deficiency.

— Zinc —

Zinc acts primarily through the role of enzymes. Zinc is required for the activity of the powerful anti-inflammatory, antioxidant enzyme super oxide dismutase (SOD). Zinc plays a major role in 25 different enzymatic systems involved in digestion and metabolism. Zinc is part of the molecular structure of 80 or more known enzymes that work with red blood cells to move carbon dioxide from tissues to lungs. Overall, zinc is a vital component of more than 200 enzymes.

— What Zinc Does in the Body —

Zinc is required for skin beauty, cell and bodily growth, sexual development, fertility, night vision, and for improving one's sense of taste and smell. It promotes cell division, cell repair, cell growth, and the production of T-lymphocyte white blood cells. It helps the lymphatic organs and the liver eliminate wastes properly. It works through the lymphatic system to help with tissue repair and oxygenation. Zinc is present in insulin and helps balance blood sugar challenges.

Zinc works synergistically with vitamins. Zinc, in combination with vitamin A and sulfur, builds strong hair.

Zinc and vitamin E (*abundant in tocotrienols, olives, and olive oil*) are necessary for the health of the reproductive system in both sexes. It is an especially important mineral for the prostate, which concentrates zinc up to 2,000% above what is found in the blood. Zinc is present in male sexual fluids. Zinc increases male potency and sex drive. Properly nourished sexual organs raise sexual energy, creating more attractiveness and appeal.

Zinc is essential for a great skin complexion because zinc is a key member of a group of enzymes that helps the body maintain its collagen supply. Without zinc, the enzymes that digest damaged collagen and rebuild new collagen do not function properly. In this way it also helps heal burns. It can even play a role in repairing DNA damage due to viruses, exposure to x-rays, and radiation. And it prevents wrinkling, stretch marks, and the outward signs of aging. Topical zinc (*zinc oxide*) preparations have long been noted to have an anti-inflammatory effect.

Best Plant Sources of Zinc
(all of these must be eaten raw)

- Poppy seeds
- Pumpkins seeds
- Pecans
- Cashews
- Pine nuts
- Macadamia nuts
- Sunflower seeds
- Sesame seeds
- Coconuts
- Spinach
  (depending on the quality of the soil)

Best Zinc Supplements

- Angstrom-sized Zinc
  (*water-soluble in a liquid dropper*)

Signs of a Zinc Deficiency Include

- Acne
- Loss of taste and smell
- Slow growth in children
- Alopecia (*hair loss*)
- Rashes
- Skin disorders
- Sterility
- Low sperm count
- Delayed wound healing
- Delayed bone maturation
- Decreased size of testicles
- Poor eyesight

— Zinc Overdose —

Zinc supplements may produce toxic symptoms if taken for a prolonged period at a dosage of over 150 mg daily. If it is acquired from food, as recommended in this book, toxic overdoses are not possible.

Signs and Symptoms of a Zinc Overdose

- A decrease of copper in blood
- Drowsiness
- Lethargy
- Light-headedness
- Difficulty with writing
- Restlessness
- Vomiting

Iron

Iron is the most active element in the human system; therefore, it needs to be renewed frequently.

Iron-rich blood produces a soft glowing tint of beauty visible just underneath the skin. Iron-rich blood is the source of magnetism (*charisma*). Notice the waning beauty of the anemic.

— What Iron Does in the Body —

In plants and animals, iron serves several distinct purposes.

Hemoglobin and chlorophyll are essentially identical. Iron is at the center of the hemoglobin molecule, just as magnesium is at the center of the identical chlorophyll molecule. Scientists studying how magnesium is switched for iron once it has been ingested have been unable to determine when the switch is made. This has led several scientists to conclude that no switch is being made at all. Essentially, they are saying that magnesium is somehow turned into iron.

Iron is found in many dark-green vegetables and herbs. Because iron from plant sources is best absorbed in the presence of vitamin C and strong stomach acid, it is a great idea to use lemons *(high in vitamin C and an excellent stimulator of stomach acid)* in preference to vinegar in green salads as part of the dressing. However, this does not discount the importance of using apple cider vinegar when desired or needed.

Iron assists the process of respiration. It is iron-rich hemoglobin in the blood that carries oxygen throughout the body. Two-thirds of the iron in the body is found in the blood. *(The remaining third is distributed in the marrow of the bones, the liver, and principally in the spleen).*

Iron generates a magnetic blood current and an electro-magnetic induction current in the nerve spirals, which pass through the walls of the arteries and veins and help build and nourish tissues.

An iron deficiency creates a low-level of oxygenation in the blood. This manifests in the form of light-headedness, weakness, and fatigue, coupled with an intolerance to cold. In relation to this, we must note that sometimes the body will purposefully keep iron levels low to help flush out parasites. This happens many times when one switches from a meat-based diet to a raw-food vegetarian diet. Also, the body takes time to adapt from heme iron sources in meat to non-heme iron

sources in plants — another reason why transition should occur at an appropriate pace. Even so, studies show that 57% of the meat-eating population is deficient in iron.

The Best Iron-Rich Foods

- Jerusalem artichokes *(sun-chokes)*
- Onions
- Burdock root
- Cacao nibs or Cacao beans *(raw chocolate)*
- Cherries
- Blackberries
- Collards
- Young lettuces
- Nettles
- Parsley
- Shallots
- Spinach
- Young Swiss chard
- Grasses
- Most dark green-leafy vegetables
- Most red-colored berries
- Sea vegetables *(dulse, nori, or kelp)*

Manganese and Iron

Manganese plays a role in the formation of cartilage, bone, and connective tissue. In particular it is involved in the formation of the cartilage shields at the ends of the bones.

Manganese and iron possess similar qualities. Manganese is contained in red blood corpuscles. It improves the oxygenation of the blood, nerves, and brain cells — it is a "giver" of oxygen. The manganese compound (MnO_2) and iron *(Fe)* are nearly identical in their properties. The word "manganese" comes from the Latin word, "magnes," meaning magnet *(due to its iron-like magnetic qualities).*

Both manganese and iron are necessary in the growth of plants.

Manganese, like zinc, is a major component of enzymes, including the incredible antioxidant, anti-inflammatory enzyme super oxide dismutase (SOD).

Manganese, we have discovered, is the iron regulator. It is biologically transmutated into iron as the body requires it. The secret of iron-rich blood is a diet rich in iron and in manganese.

Manganese is present in seeds. Upon sprouting seeds, this element is converted to become iron in the growing shoots. In his book, *Biological Transmutations*, C.L. Kervran mentions studies by Professor Baranger describing that the enzyme synthesized at the start of germination is capable of transmutating manganese into iron, and in some legume seeds transmutes 25 times the weight of manganese into iron. *(This result was achieved by adding a soluble manganese salt to distilled water).*

Because the body has an easier time intaking iron than excreting it, iron supplements may be damaging. If one is low in iron, one should ingest green vegetable juices and, if necessary, take manganese supplements.

Best Manganese Supplements

- Angstrom-sized Manganese
  (water-soluble in a liquid dropper)

Sources of Manganese

- Cloves
- Sea vegetables *(dulse, nori, or kelp)*
- Cacao beans *(raw chocolate)*
- Spinach
- Hemp seeds
- Brazil nuts
  (also high in the antioxidant mineral selenium)
- Almonds
- Pecans
- Watercress
- Kale
- Beet leaves
- Raisins
- Prunes
- Sweet potatoes
- Wild lettuces
- Many unsprouted seeds and some nuts
- Some dark green-leafy vegetables
  (such as arugula and collard greens)
- Some root vegetables

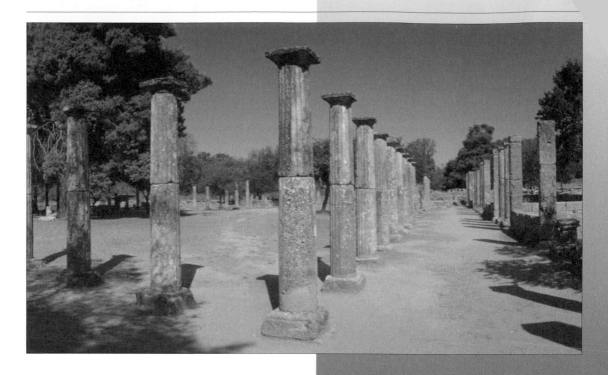

*"Inner Beauty
Creates
Outer Beauty."*

Recall from the Introduction...

"The major theme is that physical beauty is a function of inner cleanliness; it is a function of having healthy skin, hair, nails, and internal connective tissue elastically-grown from ideal raw-foods containing high concentrations of the minerals sulfur, silicon, zinc, iron and manganese. Maintaining the proper acid/alkaline pH balance in the body is a major element of this book. Another theme involves becoming parasite-free by eating foods and herbs that flush out parasites. Raw antioxidant compounds and foods *(especially those containing vitamins A, C and E) that help delay or slow free radical damage to cells and tissues (thus creating lasting youth)* are thematically referenced. Natural anti-inflammatory foods and food compounds that prevent or reverse facial puffiness are also thematically mentioned throughout these pages."

To clarify and summarize the importance of the themes in this book, the beautifying foods all possess one or more of the following qualities:

- High concentrations of the minerals sulfur, silicon, zinc, iron, and/or manganese.

- An alkaline reaction in the body.

- Anti-parasitical effects.

- High levels of antioxidants *(especially vitamins A, C, and E)*.

- Anti-inflammatory properties.

The beautifying foods cultivate a renewed charm and charisma. They add to one's inner outer beauty. Mineral-rich, nutrient-dense beauty foods are nature's best cosmetics.

This list of beautifying foods is by no means complete. The beautifying properties of foods are always being discovered. Other foods may be added later; this list represents my current understanding of beauty foods.

Aloe Vera

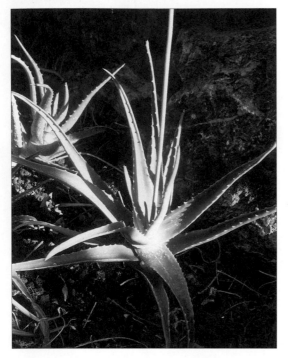

Aloe vera is a perennial succulent that likely originated in the tropics of Africa and was transferred to the western hemisphere in the 16th century. It grows in a wide range of climates and seems to do best in tropical and sub-tropical conditions. In temperate climates it grows best indoors as a houseplant.

Legend has it that Cleopatra attributed her great beauty to the practice of massaging fresh aloe vera gel onto her skin each day. Another legend describes that Alexander the Great invaded Egypt and Africa in order to capture aloe vera, which he believed to be a food of perpetual youth and rapid healing. Aloe was used by the Greeks and Romans to help quickly heal wounds.

Another legendary story indicates that the Essenes living in the area of the Dead Sea during and before the time of the Roman Empire grew exceptionally powerful aloe vera using dead sea salts and their extracts as part of their growth medium. I have personally done this and the results have been extraordinary.

Fresh aloe vera gel, when applied topically, assists in the healing of sunburns and other burns faster than any other substance. This is probably due to the high concentration of MSM *(methyl-sulfonyl-methane)* and polysaccharides that aloe vera contains.

Aloe gel is also helpful with dry skin conditions. Undoubtedly, it is the best emollient on earth. When rubbed into the face, it provides a "face-lift" in 30 minutes as the skin seems to be pulled tighter with more firmness.

The anti-inflammatory action of aloe vera in acute inflammation is one of its best known actions. It contains plant steroids and salicylic acid *(a close relative of aspirin)*, which help exert the anti-inflammatory effect.

— How To Use Aloe Vera —
Each leaf should be sliced and filleted to expose the healing inner gel. The gel may then be eaten or used topically as a "lotion."

To create a wonderful beauty tonic, blend the gel with orange or papaya juice.

— How To Select Aloe Vera —
Select aloe vera that is juicy and plump with gel. The larger leaves tend to be easier to use. My experience has been that aloe with a yellower gel has greater skin-tightening effects.

Preferentially choose outdoor aloe vera as it will retain a high concentration of MSM absorbed from rain.

Arugula
Arugula *(also known as Rocket in the United Kingdom)* is a Mediterranean-type of cruciferous green-leafy vegetable that grows so pervasively in the wild that it was not cultivated until recent years. The leaves are somewhat

dandelion-like in shape, and have an appetizing, yet spicy flavor that is peppery and reminiscent of other foods in the mustard family. Like watercress, arugula is more rich than a typical green-leafy vegetable, yet less rich than a strong herb. Still widely used as a salad green in southern Europe, arugula has quickly grown popular in health-food stores all across North America.

Arugula has a strong, spicy flavor. It is seemingly eaten by more women than men, earning it the title of the "queen of the cruciferous vegetables."

— Nutrition —

Arugula is highly alkaline and neutralizes acidic waste products throughout the blood and lymphatic system.

As a cruciferous vegetable, arugula ranks high in sulfur and beta-carotene *(vitamin A)*.

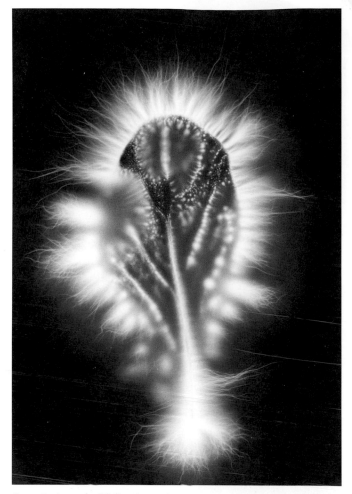

Organic Arugula *(Kirlian Image)*

The cruciferous vegetables are one of the best sources of beta-carotene. This is beneficial because beta-carotene protects the nucleus of each cell from radiation. Thus, it protects the skin from sun damage. Beta-carotene also helps to inhibit acne. It helps fight topical infections and cancer. In combination with zinc and sulfur, beta-carotene creates healthy hair.

Arugula also contains: dithiolthiones, a group of anti-cancer and antioxidant substances; indoles, a group of substances that protect against colon and breast cancer; and, of course, sulfurous mustard oils that have beautifying, as well as antibiotic and antiviral, effects.

Because of its high sulfur content, arugula is an excellent internal skin cleanser and liver purifier.

— How To Select Arugula —

When selecting arugula in the store, look for strong, vigorous, fresh-picked bunches. Avoid weak or wilted leaves.

Arugula is easy to grow and tastes best when picked before the plant flowers and goes to seed. To harvest arugula, simply pick the young leaves and the plant will keep regrowing new ones for months. Older leaves are a bit tougher and spicier. Drought-affected plants will typically be smaller and spicier.

I urge you to seek out wild arugula whenever possible. I particularly enjoy the wild arugula growing all over North America.

— How To Eat Arugula —

Arugula makes an excellent addition to any salad. Arugula combines well with other green vegetables.

If you can get them, pick up some arugula flowers. They are small *(the size of a fingernail)*, broccoli-like, and may be used in salads for a light, peppery flavor.

Mixing arugula in a salad with avocados and olive oil tends to calm the leaves' spicy elements.

Burdock Root

Burdock probably originated in Siberia. It now grows all over the world as a common weed. The root of this plant is somewhat like a carrot, yet more mucilaginous, thinner in shape, and a bit juicier *(especially when picked fresh)*. The root is brown on the outside and white on the inside.

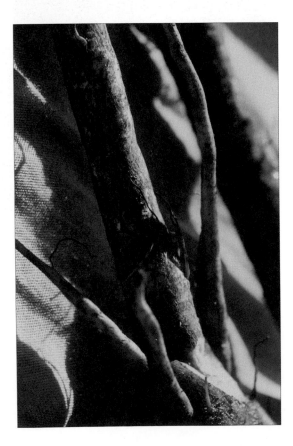

Burdock root has been traditionally used in Ayurvedic medicine *(the ancient healing system of India)* to alleviate skin challenges such as rashes, acne, abscesses, local skin infections, eczema, and psoriasis. Ayurvedic philosophy considers burdock root to be one of nature's great skin cleansers and best blood purifiers.

Burdock root is also part of the Native American derived, cancer-fighting Essiac tea formula. Advocates of this formula *(of which I am one)* generally regard Burdock root as one of nature's best blood purifiers.

Burdock root is very concentrated in both vitamins *(B1, B2, B3, C)* and in beauty minerals *(iron, manganese, silicon, and zinc)*. It is balanced between quantities of calcium and phosphorous, making it neutral in pH *(a good characteristic for a root, as most roots, such as the potato, are acid-forming)*.

Herbalists often talk of the Doctrine of Signatures *(through which foods look, feel, and taste like what they heal)*. The taste of burdock is almost slightly metallic, like blood, indicating its efficacy in that area. Its phallic shape indicates aphrodisiac qualities. In China, burdock is considered an aphrodisiac.

I consider burdock root an excellent beautifier of the teeth. This characteristic probably corresponds to its brilliant white inner flesh. It also correlates with its high mineral content.

Burdock root is a nonsteroidal, anti-inflammatory food. It is great for inflammatory conditions, especially those associated with psoriasis.

Burdock root improves digestion, stimulates digestive juices, increases bile flow, and increases kidney function. Burdock root contains the compound inulin, which is a great food source for probiotics *(friendly intestinal bacteria)*.

The leaves of the burdock plant can be mashed and applied to stings produced by stinging nettles. This will alleviate the sting in minutes.

I usually recommend that people start acclimating to the taste of burdock root by including it in their fresh juices. It is different and actually tastes quite good. A good juice to start with is:

Apple, Celery, Burdock Root Juice

2 apples

4 ribs of celery

1 burdock root.

Run all ingredients through a juicer.

— How To Select Burdock Root —

Select burdock roots that are crisp and somewhat stiff. If burdock is flimsy, it has lost its vitality.

For those who have a garden, burdock root is easy to grow, especially in temperate climates. If you grow your own burdock and have an excess, you can thinly slice and dry the roots. These dried roots can be powdered and eaten, or they may utilized for teas.

Coconuts and Coconut Oil
— Young Coconuts —

Coconut palms are prehistoric plants that are distantly related to grasses. In Sanskrit *(the language of ancient India)*, the coconut palm is known as "kalpa vriksha" meaning "the tree that supplies all that is needed to live."

Exactly where coconut palms originated is unknown, but a few scholars in this field suggest it was the Philippines. The Philippines have the densest population of coconut palm trees of anywhere I have personally visited and seen.

Coconuts can survive many months floating at sea. As described by Plato, coconuts existed in ancient Atlantis. They were carried by ancient mariners throughout the world.

Elaborate computer simulations of ocean currents and drift show that humans had to carry coconuts to America. They were on the southwest coast of Mexico when the Spanish arrived there, and coconuts palms were cultivated in all Mayan lands.

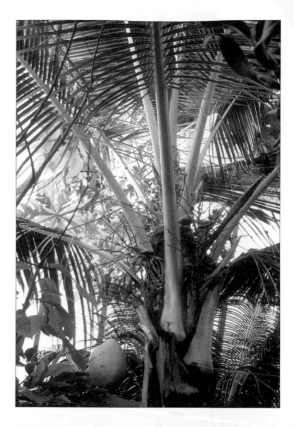

"Moreover, there was a great number of elephants in the island…and the fruits having a hard rind, affording drinks…All these things they received from the earth, and they employed themselves in constructing their temples, palaces, harbors, and docks."

— *Plato, describing coconuts on the lost continent of Atlantis*

— Coconuts Can Save Your Life —

Coconuts are one of the greatest gifts on this planet. No matter where you are, what you have done, how much you have mistreated your body, fresh young coconuts and coconut oil can save your life.

The coconut is a natural water filter that takes almost nine months to filter each liter *(quart)* of water in the shell. To get there, the water levitates upward through innumerable fibers that purify it before it ends up in the sterile nut. This clear coconut water is

...ur the highest sources of electrolytes found in nature.

Young coconut water is identical to human blood plasma, making it the universal donor. Plasma makes up 55% of human blood. The remaining 45% of our blood consists of hemoglobin, which is essentially transformed plant blood *(chlorophyll)*. When we consume a drink consisting of 55% fresh coconut water and 45% fresh green-leaf juice, we give ourselves an instant blood transfusion.

Coconuts in their young stage of growth are the most health enhancing. In their youth, they contain a soft "spoon meat." This meat consists mostly of a pure, raw saturated fat. This soft "spoon meat" has the most remarkable ability to rejuvenate oxidative tissue damage, improve the functioning of the nervous system, and restore male sexual fluids.

Whenever we are in tropical countries, we should drink and eat at least three or four young coconuts each day. In North America and Europe, young Thai coconuts are available in Asian markets. These are not as optimal as the wild tropical coconuts *(e.g. growing in Hawaii and Mexico)*, but are still quite good and work especially well as a base for smoothies.

Thai coconuts, like most imported coconuts, have been shaved down from their original size and shape. In Asian markets, these plastic-wrapped young white coconuts are easy to recognize because they are flat on one side, cylindrical around the edges, and conical on top. When purchasing these, seek out the newest coconuts that have come into the market. Any mold or moisture underneath the plastic indicates that the nut is spoiled.

The brown, hairy coconuts most people are familiar with are mature coconuts. They can contain a good quality of coconut water *(not always)*, yet the flesh is hard and fibrous, unlike the soft meat of the youthful stage. The fibrous and protein-rich meat is less tasty and not as digestible, even though it contains one of the most healing fat substances yet known.

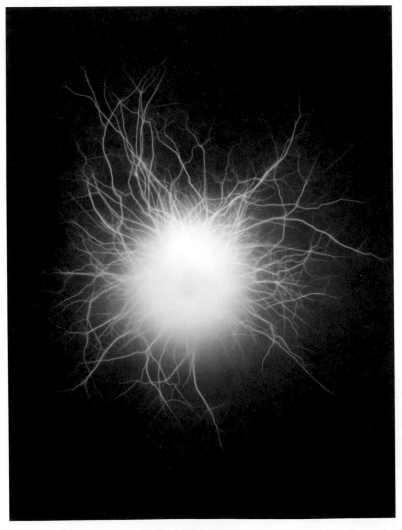

A Drop of Raw Organic Coconut Oil (*Kirlian Image*)

Select brown hairy coconuts by looking at the three holes on one side of the coconut. If there is mold on any of the three holes, select another one. Choose coconuts free of mold.

Coconut Oil

The challenge with mature coconuts is that they contain a high quantity of coarse protein and fiber *(three times as much fiber as vegetables)* which surrounds the nourishing, cleansing coconut oil. This is solved by cold-pressing the healing fat/oil out of the fiber, thus concentrating its essence into a butter.

Coconut oil *(sometimes called coconut butter)* is derived from mature coconuts containing hardened white flesh. The white flesh is shredded and collected. In a cold-pressing process, the shredded coconut is pressed at 90-100 degrees Fahrenheit *(32-38 degrees Celsius)*. The oil is melted, pressed out, and collected to create a concentrated essence of coconut called coconut oil.

For clarity, there is no major difference between a fat and an oil; the terms are used interchangeably. However, in the way I use the words, a fat remains a solid at room temperature, while an oil remains a liquid at room temperature. Coconut oil and coconut butter are actually the same thing. Creamy white coconut butter becomes a clear oil when it is warmed above 78 degrees Fahrenheit *(26 degrees Celsius)*. When in a liquid form, it is called coconut oil.

Coconut oil has been used as a food and medicine since the dawn of history. Ayurveda *(the medicine of India)* and the medicinal systems of Polynesia have long advocated its therapeutic and cosmetic properties.

Unlike the high-calorie, cholesterol-soaked, long-chain, saturated animal fats found in meat and dairy products, coconut oil is a raw saturated fat containing mostly medium-chain fatty acids that the body can metabolize efficiently and convert to energy quickly. By weight, coconut oil has less calories than any other fat source.

— Medium Chain Fatty Acids — *(MCFAs)*

Fats are chains of carbon atoms *(of varying lengths)* surrounded by various quantities of hydrogen. The arrangement of hydrogen around a carbon chain determines its saturation. The more hydrogen, the more saturation and the more stable the molecule.

The length of the carbon chain in fat determines many of its properties. Coconut oil is a saturated fat, but it consists primarily of medium chain fatty acids *(MCFAs)* of 8 to 12 carbon atoms in length. Some saturated fatty acids in meats, for example, range in length from 14 to 24 carbon atoms while some of those in urine, butter, and vinegar range in length from 2 to 6 carbon atoms in length.

The MCFAs in coconut oil possess incredible health-giving properties.

The shorter MCFA chains require less energy and fewer enzymes to digest. In most people, coconut oil can be emulsified during digestion without burdening the liver or gall bladder. Thus, coconut oil provides more energy, more quickly than other fat sources. Many individuals who suffer from poor digestion — and especially liver or gall bladder trouble — would benefit from eating coconut oil rather than other oils.

— MCFA — Immune System Enhancing Properties

Coconut oil contains the following MCFAs:

- Caprylic acid *(C-8)*
- Capric acid *(C-10)*
- Lauric acid *(C-12)*
- Myristic acid *(C-14)*

All these demonstrate anti-viral, anti-microbial, and anti-fungal properties. Lauric acid has the greatest anti-viral activity. Caprylic acid is the most potent yeast-fighting substance.

MCFAs disrupt the lipid membranes of viruses, bacteria, yeast, and fungi. Lipid-coated viruses and bacteria contain lipids in their membranes that are similar to those in

MCFAs confuse microbes and virus- because they can no longer calibrate the location of their membranes in the presence of coconut oil. This causes them to spill their genetic contents and become easy prey for white blood cells to consume.

Those who suffer from candida or other fungal conditions can benefit from coconut oil. Some forms of psoriasis are actually skin infections caused by a fungus. These can be helped by using coconut oil topically.

— Cholesterol —

Most pieces of information relating to saturated fat and cholesterol circulating in the mass media are inaccurate. Saturated fats have been the target of a host of hostile propaganda. This propaganda claims that saturated fats lead to clogging of the arteries, when, in reality, arterial plaque is nearly 75% cooked unsaturated fat and foreign cholesterol (derived from eating animal products).

Coconut oil contains no cholesterol and actually helps to lower cholesterol levels. It outperforms cold-pressed olive oil in this regard. People from coconut-eating cultures in the tropics have consistently lower cholesterol levels than people in the U.S.

The cholesterol-lowering properties of coconut oil are a direct result of its ability to stimulate thyroid function. In the presence of adequate thyroid hormone, cholesterol (specifically LDL-cholesterol) is converted by enzymatic processes to necessary anti-aging steroids, progesterone, DHEA, and pregnenolone. These substances are required to help prevent heart disease, senility, obesity, cancer, and other diseases associated with aging and degeneration.

In his books, Dr. Raymond Peat (a leading researcher in the field of hormones) details that coconut oil, when added regularly to a balanced diet, lowers cholesterol to normal by promoting its conversion into pregnenolone. Pregnenolone is also the precursor to many hormones including progesterone. Dr. Peat recommends increasing one's pregnenolone levels for women with hormone imbalances.

Pregnenolone is a major factor that gives coconut oil its beautifying qualities. Pregnenolone improves circulation in the skin, gives the face a lift, restores sagging skin, and reduces bags under the eyes by promoting the contractions of muscle-like cells. Pregnenolone counters fatigue, enhances the memory, protects the nerves from stress, and has anti-anxiety properties.

— Antioxidants —

As a derivative of coconut oil, pregnenolone is an antioxidant. Dr. Peat theorizes that coconut oil itself may also have antioxidant properties, since the oil is highly stable and it reduces our need for vitamin E, whereas unsaturated oils deplete vitamin E.

Research findings indicate that coconut oil appears to double the body's ability to use antioxidant, omega 3 fatty acids. Because of this, I recommend that individuals take omega 3 containing oils (flax seed oil, hempseed oil, krill oil, fish oil, etc.) with coconut oil.

— Blood Sugar —

For those of us who use coconut oil consistently, one of the most noticeable changes is the ability to go for several hours without eating, and to feel hungry without having symptoms of hypoglycemia and erratic blood-sugar levels. Erratic blood sugar swings stress the system, calling in the use of the adrenal glands (low blood sugar is a signal for the release of adrenal hormones).

Shifting to coconut oil as a fat source normalizes bloods sugar levels, increases energy, decreases the stress on our system, and thus reduces our need for the adrenal hormones. Removing the effects of adrenal stress alleviates dark circles from around the eyes.

— The Thyroid Gland — and Weight Loss

Dr. Peat describes that in the 1940s, farmers attempted to use coconut oil to fatten their animals, yet they found it made the animals lean and active. This was not the effect they were looking for. They wanted to fatten their animals for slaughter and thus, within ten years, chose to give their animals soy and corn feed. Soy and corn feed slow the thyroid, causing animals to get fat without eating much food.

Cooked unsaturated oils *(derived from seeds such as: corn oil, safflower oil, canola oil, soy margarine, etc.)* suppress the metabolism, contributing to hypothyroidism *(and weight gain)*. This occurs because cooked unsaturated oils not only suppress our tissue's response to the thyroid hormone, but also suppress the transport of the hormone on the thyroid-transport protein.

Consuming coconut oil regularly restores thyroid function, often helps relieve hypothyroidism, and actually increases the metabolic rate leading to weight loss.

Those who are taking artificial thyroid medication must be cautious in coming off that drug. Thyroid medication strongly influences metabolism. Please consult with your holistic physician if you undergo a program to wean yourself from thyroid medication.

— Skin —

After a bottle of unsaturated oil *(corn oil, safflower oil, canola oil, soy margarine, etc.)* has been opened several times, a few drops typically dribble onto the outside of the bottle. These drops become very sticky and difficult to wash off. Once inside the body this characteristic of rancid oil leads to wrinkles, "liver spots" in the skin, and lesions in the brain, heart, blood vessels, eyes, etc. As cooked unsaturated oil increases in the diet, the rate of oxidative damage increases, leading to aged, damaged skin.

Repairing and nourishing the skin with coconut oil should be approached by both eating coconut oil and massaging it into the skin.

Coconut oil reverses the tissue-damaging process by displacing cooked oil from the tissues and providing fat-soluble vitamins, minerals, and supernutrition factors *(i.e. pregnenolone)* directly to the damaged tissue.

Coconut oil has been used as a skin moisturizer for thousands of years. It is ideal for dry, rough, and wrinkled skin. Because it consists mostly of MCFAs, it is easily absorbed by the skin. It prevents stretch marks and lightens existing ones. It is an excellent lip balm. Its antiseptic elements keep the skin young and healthy and relatively free from infections. All these factors make coconut oil ideal for massage and massage therapists.

Rancid fats and oils found in everyday commercial lotions and creams are absorbed through the skin and negatively affect the connective tissues. They provide temporary relief from dry skin, but eventually weaken the skin over time. Generally, the more standard commercial lotions and creams that one uses, the worse the skin becomes.

In his book, *The Coconut Oil Miracle*, Bruce Fife, N.D. details: "Studies show that dry skin contains a higher content of unsaturated fatty acids *(60%)* compared to normal skin *(49%)*. The best oil to use is one that doesn't create free radicals. Saturated fats fit that requirement."

I use Sunfood Nutrition's Organic Coconut Oil as an essential lotion. I use this coconut oil after sunbathing to help create and hold on to a beautiful tan. I often bring a bottle with me when I do large seminars and lectures. Before going on stage, I rub some into my hands, face, neck, even my gums. It has a pleasant odor and provides a certain radiance in the skin.

— Sunfood Nutrition's Coconut Oil —

As with any oil, all coconut butter/oil that you use should be cold-pressed and packaged in dark glass bottles. All butters and oils are light-sensitive. Sunfood Nutrition's Coconut Oil is sealed in dark amber glass containers to keep damaging spectrums of light from reaching the oil.

Sunfood Nutrition's Organic Coconut Oil is very stable and can be kept in a cupboard at room temperature. It can be refrigerated after opening, but this is not required to ensure freshness. It can remain stable for over two years and some people suggest five years with proper storage *(no light, heat, or oxygen)*.

..., *The Coconut Oil Miracle*, Bruce
..., N.D., tells us: "According to Leigh
Broadhurst, Ph.D., a scientist at the USDA
Human Nutrition Research Center in
Beltville, Maryland, saturated fatty acids are
300 or more times more resistant to oxidation
than alpha-linolenic acid *(flaxseed oil)*. In other
words, coconut oil will remain fresh 300
times longer than flaxseed oil. For instance, to
equal the amount of oxidative damage that
occurs in flaxseed oil in just 30 minutes of
processing, coconut oil would have to be sub-
jected to the same conditions for 150 continuous hours — that's over six days."

— How To Eat Coconut Oil —

Coconut oil can be used as a food. It can be
eaten straight, blended into a salad dressing,
or mixed into a smoothie *(if Sun Is Shining
Superfood is also added, this makes an excellent
drink)*. The recommended daily intake is one
to four tablespoons *(a therapeutic dose consists
of at least three tablespoons daily)*.

— Coconut Oil As An Erotic Oil —

Coconut oil is a great erotic oil. The smell
and taste of this oil enhance sexual inter-
course. Its anti-viral, anti-microbial properties also provide some *(although not complete)*
protection from sexually-transmitted diseases (STDs). For long-term monogamous
relationships, coconut oil is a great choice.
For new relationships, condoms and other
appropriate protection from STDs should be
used. Coconut oil should be used with
polyurethane condoms or a natural skin con-
dom. Latex condoms should not be used,
because coconut oil can dissolve latex.

— Cooking —

I promote raw-food nutrition. At the same
time, there must be ample opportunity to
transition and to offer friends and family,
who are momentarily lacking interest in raw-
foods, healthy alternatives. One of the greatest pieces of information one could derive
from this book is to only and exclusively use
coconut oil for all cooking needs. Coconut
butter/oil is the most stable *(of any known
butter/oil)* at high temperatures *(up to 170*

degrees Fahrenheit). Therefore, if one is going
to heat or cook any food, coconut butter/oil
should be the only butter/oil ever used. This
means using coconut oil for cooking in place
of butter, margarine, olive oil, canola oil, corn
oil, safflower oil, etc. Unlike all these
fats/oils, coconut oil does not form dangerous
trans-fatty acids because it is a completely
saturated fat.

Cucumbers

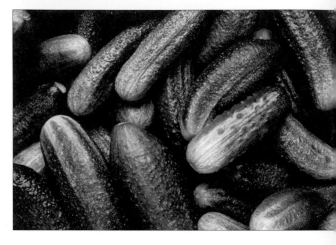

Cucumbers are a prominent member of the
melon family. They are unique as a melon
due to their high-water content and low
sugar content. They are native to western
Asia and were a popular vegetable-fruit
amongst the ancient Egyptians, Sumerians,
Greeks, and Romans. Many cultures considered them a symbol of fertility. Alexander the
Great introduced the cucumber into Europe.
Christopher Columbus introduced them to
the Americas.

Cucumbers have a reputation as the best
kidney cleanser known. They are a diuretic;
thus, they prevent bloating due to water
retention, and they help to wash the kidneys
and bladder of debris and stones.

Cucumbers mix well with celery in a juice.
The natural saltiness of the celery helps to
transport the water-rich cucumber juice into
the tissues, creating more hydration. One of
the most beautifying and cleansing of all

juices combines celery, apple, and cucumber together in the following ratio:

- 4-6 ribs of celery
- 1 apple
- 1 cucumber

Cucumbers contain the enzyme erepsin, which helps to digest proteins, kill tapeworms, and support healthy kidneys.

The shininess of cucumber skins is indicative of the presence of silicon. Waxing and the usage of pesticides cause most people to skin their cucumbers before eating them. The best idea is to buy fresh organic cucumbers. This way you can eat the skins and enjoy the benefits of the beautifying silicon compounds and chlorophyll present there.

Cucumbers have been the favorite food of dieters for thousands of years. The Roman Emperor Tiberius was said to enjoy cucumbers so much that he ate 10 of them each day. Cucumbers are cooling, refreshing, water-rich, filling, low in calories, alkaline, and high in energy. Many of the world's most attractive actresses and models eat cucumbers daily.

Ideally cucumbers should be chosen ripe, when they are plump, firm, and medium green to slightly yellow in color.

Durian

Durian is the most exotic and sensual of all Southeast Asian fruits. It grows throughout Vietnam, Indochina, Thailand, the Philippines, Malaysia, and Indonesia. It has also been introduced to and is growing in Brazil, Honduras, Costa Rica, Hawaii, and Puerto Rico. Durians grow only in tropical climates on a jungle tree that can exceed 30 meters *(100 feet)* in height!

Durian is the favorite food of orangutans, elephants, tigers, and all other jungle creatures who know of its existence. When durian trees produce flowers, fruit bats feed almost exclusively on their nectar.

The strong, pungent odor of durian is ecstatic to some, nearly nauseating to others. Until one tastes this fruit, all judgment should be withheld. Once someone is hooked on the flavor of durian, the interesting smell all but disappears.

"Its consistence and flavour are indescribable. A rich butterlike custard highly flavoured with almonds gives the best general idea of it, but intermingled with it come wafts of flavours that call to mind cream cheese, onion sauce, brown sherry, and other incongruities. Then there is a rich glutinous smoothness in the pulp which nothing else possesses, but which adds to its delicacy. It is neither acid nor sweet or juicy, yet one feels the want of none of these qualities, for it is perfect as it is. It produces no nausea or other bad effect, and the more you eat of it the less you feel inclined to stop. In fact to eat durians is a new sensation, worth a voyage to the East to experience."

— *Alfred Russell Wallace, Famous Naturalist, The Malay Archipelago*

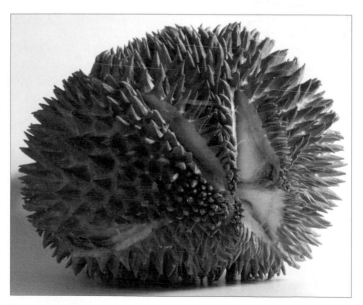

Organic Durian

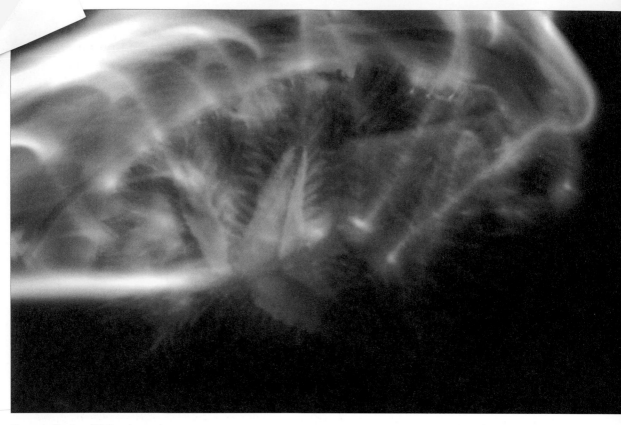

Organic Durian (*Kirlian Image*)

Ancient Burmese kings had runners carry durians over 150 kilometers *(80 miles)* to their courts.

The durian fruit is one of largest tree fruits in the world. The fruit grows to be the size of a large oblong honeydew melon, and can weigh over 4 kilograms *(10 pounds)*. The fruit is a capsule that contains five to six sections containing edible "pillows." Around the inner edible "pillows" is a thick, bone-like, skin-shell structure with sharp spines surrounding the exterior of the fruit. The spines are so sharp that people are killed every year in Asia by falling durians.

Durians contain high levels of tryptophan. This is an amino acid and a tryptamine *(similar to serotonin, melatonin, and DMT)*. Researchers have discovered that tryptophan helps anxious, depressed, repressed people, as well as insomniacs. Tryptophan works by raising serotonin levels in the brain and nervous system. When serotonin levels increase, a euphoric feeling is felt as a free passage is cleared for nerve impulses to travel.

Durians are such a strong blood cleanser that eating a few durians a day can change the odor of one's urine *(urine is filtered out of blood)*.

What gives durians their strongest beautifying characteristics is their high concentration of raw oleic fats *(and vitamin E)*, sulfur compounds, and soft proteins. Durians actually contain one of the highest concentrations of protein of any fruit, making them an excellent muscle builder.

Those who eat durians are known to be more attractive. According to Singapore lore, "when the durians come down from the trees, the sarongs come off." This is in reference to the durian's legendary powers as an attractor and an aphrodisiac.

Durians are available in many North American and European Asian markets in frozen, dried, or fresh form. Fresh durians are more rare, yet tastier, have a more pleasant texture and contain more of the nutrient value than those that have been frozen. Dried durians are quite extraordinary.

How To Select Durians

When choosing a frozen durian, look for three characteristics:

1. Choose browner and yellower durians instead of green.

2. Choose a durian that is just starting to split its skin longitudinally.

3. Choose durians that are heavier for their size.

When choosing fresh durians, purchase them just as they begin to split longitudinally. Look to see that the stem has been cleanly cut. If the fruit is ready to eat then, when you shake it, you should be able to hear the fruit pillows moving inside. Ask the seller if they are willing to open the durian for you (*to see if it is a good one*). They will continue to ripen and split if left at room temperature on the kitchen counter. When they begin to smell strongly, they are ready to eat. To eat the fruit, split open the shell and eat the golden pillows.

Figs

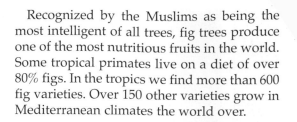

Recognized by the Muslims as being the most intelligent of all trees, fig trees produce one of the most nutritious fruits in the world. Some tropical primates live on a diet of over 80% figs. In the tropics we find more than 600 fig varieties. Over 150 other varieties grow in Mediterranean climates the world over.

The Roman historian, Aeliant, tells us that in the first age of humankind the "Athenians lived on figs…" (*Aeliant Hist. Var., L. 8, ch. 89*).

Figs are a densely mineralized sweet fruit. They contain one of the highest concentrations of calcium of any food.

Whether they are fresh or naturally dried, figs are a great laxative. The tiny seeds in figs are not only packed with nutrients, but they help draw out and dissolve waste, parasites, and mucus in the intestines. Figs are one of Professor Arnold Ehret's top three mucus-dissolving foods (*as referenced in The Mucusless Diet Healing System*).

Dried figs are probably the healthiest choice of all dried fruits. They are the most alkaline of dried fruits and probably the most mineral-rich as well.

— How To Eat Figs —

Fresh figs should be soft and as tree-ripened as possible. If many figs are eaten unripe, they can burn the mouth and lips. Figs are a wonderful treat by themselves, but also mix with other foods well, due to their high alkaline-mineral content.

Dried figs may be eaten by themselves; however, I typically like to blend them in smoothies in order to add

"…champions were in times past, fed with figs."

—*Pliny, Roman Naturalist*

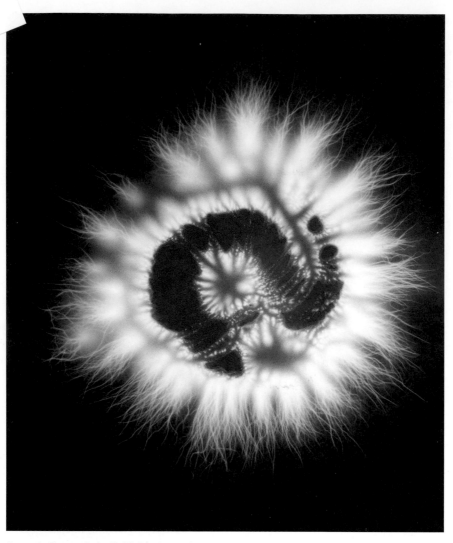

Organic Fig cut in half *(Kirlian Image)*

incredible zest and flavor. I also cut them up and mix them with salads.

— How To Select Figs —

As mentioned on the previous page, select fresh figs that are soft and as tree-ripened as you can find.

Dried Calimyrna figs are, nutritionally and by taste, the best dried fruit available.

Hemp Seed

"Make the most of the Indian hemp seed and sow it everywhere."

— *George Washington*

Hemp grows all over the world. It is believed to have first appeared on Earth somewhere between Afghanistan and the Fertile Crescent *(present-day Iraq)*. Hemp leaves and seeds were used as a food source long before the beginning of recorded history.

Hemp fiber has been used for textiles and rope since the beginning of recorded history. Hemp leaves and seeds were grown and used as food by America's founding fathers. Thomas Jefferson said that the future of America depends on the growth of this crop — hemp!

Hemp seeds are like tiny nuts that develop out of the female hemp flowers. They are small; 1,000 hemp seeds may weigh as little as 15 grams *(0.5 ounces).*

The taste of hemp seeds is so wonderful, and the history of their cultural use as a food so vast, that most people reconnect with this food immediately upon tasting them.

Hemp seeds are one of the most nutritionally complete foods on the planet earth. They contain all nine essential amino acids in a favorable ratio. They also contain the essential fatty acids omega 3 and omega 6, and they are heavily mineralized.

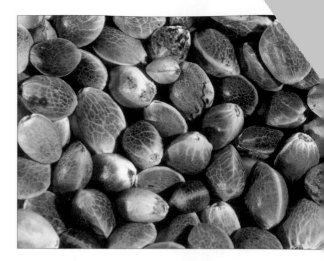

— Hemp Protein —
(Edestin)

Shelled hemp seeds consist of 36.6% protein, making them, by weight, the highest protein food on Earth, with the exception of algaes. 65+% of hemp-seed protein is in the form of globular edestin. The globular form of this protein gives hemp seeds a high protein content without the abrasiveness found in most high-protein foods. This makes hemp seeds uniquely beautifying in that they are softly, yet quickly, nourishing and strength-building.

Hemp seeds contain an important quantity of raw protein, that includes the sulfur-bearing amino acids: methionine, cysteine, and cystine. These can be immediately utilized to build strong hair, nails, skin, muscle and connective tissue. *(see Lesson 7: Alchemical Beauty Secrets).*

Many people are allergic to abrasive protein foods such as dairy, soy, whey, and beans. No allergies to hemp protein have yet been reported to me. Hemp seeds are free from trypsin inhibitors found in certain seeds, such as soybeans, that interfere with protein digestion.

Hemp seeds, along with vegetables, nuts, other seeds, and, if needed, certain algaes and/or bee pollen, can adequately supply high quantities of proteins and amino acids to allow success with a raw-food lifestyle.

"A body fed with a diet rich in quality amino acids is able to maintain the best quality of health. Collagen protein is the most abundant protein in the body and is largely dependant on a constant supply of amino acids. Collagen is often cited as the protein that provides for skin health, strength, elasticity, and beauty. Collagen actually plays a part in the health of all body tissues, from the bones and teeth to the hair and nails. It also is present in the corneas and lenses of the eyes. Those who follow a diet that is lacking in quality amino acids and essential fatty acids exhibit this in a less vibrant physical appearance, including in the skin, hair, nails, and eyes. Hemp seed provides the essential fatty acid and amino acid nutrients in the best form and at the best ratio for the body to maintain vibrant, strong, elastic, and healthy tissues."

— *John McCabe,*
   Hemp: What the World Needs Now

Hempseed Oils —

...eeds are the only food known that ...ain the exact ratio of essential fatty acids *(one part omega 3 to three parts omega 6)*. Flax seeds and flax oil provide therapeutic quantities of omega 3, yet hemp seeds provide a long-term stable source of omega 3, omega 6 *(including GLA)*, and omega 9 *(a beautifying monounsaturated fat)*.

Omega 3 fatty acids *(found in hemp seeds, hemp oil, flax seeds, and flax oil)* are essential fatty acids. They are called "essential" because they must be present in our diet to experience good health. These fatty acids are strong antioxidants. They protect us from the sun and build beautiful skin. They also strengthen the immune system and help us to burn excess fat.

Hemp seed is the highest natural source of gamma linolenic acid *(GLA)*, a type of super-omega 6 fatty acid that has strong anti-inflammatory properties. GLA also helps maintain hormonal balance.

Within unsprouted hemp seeds we find small undeveloped green leaves waiting to be sprouted, making hemp seeds one of the few unsprouted seeds that contain chlorophyll.

Hemp seeds contain a significant quantity of lecithin. This nutrient is excellent for building the internal organs *(liver, brain, etc.)*.

Because hemp is such a strong plant *(still close to its natural state)*, even non-organic hemp crops are typically not sprayed with pesticides.

— Minerals —

Hemp seeds are one of the most mineral-rich foods found on Earth. They contain the following impressive array of minerals and trace minerals *(listed in order of dominance)*:

- Phosphorous
  (an energy storage mineral)
- Potassium
  (an active energy mineral)
- Magnesium
  (builds bone and opens over 300 different detoxification pathways in the body)
- Sulfur
  (a beauty mineral)
- Calcium
  (relaxes the digestive tract and muscles)
- Iron
  (a blood-builder and an oxgenator)
- Manganese
  (a blood-builder and an oxgenator)
- Zinc
  (an immune system, adrenal, and beauty mineral)
- Sodium
  (balances potassium, feeds the adrenals)
- Silicon
  (a bone-building, beauty mineral)
- Copper
  (reverses gray hair)
- Platinum
  (an enzymatic master mineral)
- Boron
  (assists with calcium assimilation, normalizes hormones during menopause)
- Thorium
- Strontium
- Barium
- Nickel
  (plays a key role in enzyme metabolism)
- Germanium
  (sits on the end of the DNA strand)
- Tin
  (helps reverse male pattern baldness)
- Tungsten
- Titanium
- Zirconium
- Iodine
  (a thyroid mineral that reverses hypothyroidism and assists the immune system)
- Chromium
  (a pancreatic mineral)
- Silver
  (an enzymatic mineral)
- Lithium
  (an alkaline mineral)

*Note: This mineral list is derived from *Drugs Masquerading As Food* by Suzar. Comments about the minerals are provided by David Wolfe.

— THC and Hemp —

Only two to three percent of hemp varieties are considered "marijuana." This is because only those varieties have a particularly high level of THC *(delta-9-tetrahydrocannabinol)*, the psychoactive ingredient found in their leaves and flowers that creates a "high."

Nevertheless, hemp seeds and oil do contain trace amounts of THC. In its raw unheated state, THC is one of the most powerful antioxidants known. Studies suggest that a dose as high as 5 milligrams of THC causes no psychoactive effects in an individual weighing 68 kilograms *(150 pounds)*. To obtain 5 milligrams of THC from hemp seeds, one must consume 2.5 kilograms *(5 pounds)* of shelled hemp seeds *(containing 2 parts per million of THC)* in a day. Even though they taste amazing, consuming 5 pounds of them in a day would be quite a feat!

— How To Eat Hemp Seeds —

Hemp seeds are great eaten alone as a snack. They go well sprinkled on salads. They blend well and add richness and flavor to smoothies and salad dressings.

Hemp seeds may be soaked in water, if desired, to lower enzyme inhibitors typically found in seeds. I personally like to eat them plain, without soaking them in water.

— How To Select Hemp Seeds —

To be imported into the United States, hemp seeds must be cracked out of their shells *(hemp agriculture is illegal in most of the U.S., but the laws are shifting quickly because of the realized value of this incredible plant)*.

Imported hemp seeds and hemp protein products from Canada are currently available by mail order. They are also found in some healthfood stores.

Macadamia Nuts

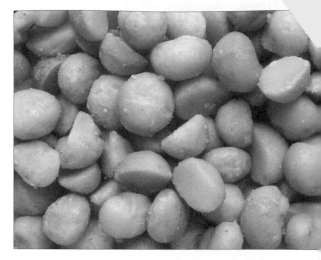

Macadamia nuts are native to southeastern Queensland and northeastern New South Wales in Australia, where they grow wild in rain forests and close to streams.

The macadamia tree was introduced into Hawaii around 1881, where it was used as an

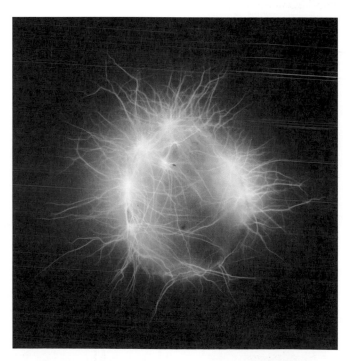

Raw Organic Macadamia Nut (*Kirlian Image*)

ree and for reforestation. The
...icultural Experiment Station
...d and introduced several promising
selections in 1948, which led to the modern
macadamia industry in Hawaii. In California
two seedling macadamias were planted in the
early 1880s, and are still standing on the cam-
pus of the University of California at Berkeley.
The importation of unique varieties into
California from Hawaii began around 1950.

Macadamia trees are also grown in South
Africa and Central America, where they produce increasingly abundant harvests.

Macadamias are ideally adapted to a mild,
frost-free climate with abundant rainfall distributed throughout the year — roughly the
same climate suitable for growing coffee.
Macadamia nuts do grow surprisingly well in
the coastal areas of California, although varieties
often respond differently to a given location.

Macadamia nuts are contained within a
hard brown shell enclosed in a green husk that
splits open as the nut matures. The brown
shell varies from smooth to bumpy depending
on variety. The nut itself is creamy white and
contains up to 80% oil and 5% carbohydrates.

Macadamia nuts were part of the
Australian aborigine's indigenous diet. They
were considered a prized delicacy and
regarded as one of nature's finest foods. The
kernels were typically consumed raw. Some
tribes extracted the oils. They used the oil as
a liniment base, as cosmetic oil, and for face
and body decorations.

Macadamias are very high in selenium, second only to Brazil nuts in that respect.
Selenium builds selenium superoxide dismutase — the body's most powerful antioxidant
enzyme. Macadamia nuts are also unusually
high in the beautifying mineral zinc.

— Fatty Acids —
It is now well established that macadamias
are an unusually rich source of healthy, beautifying oils. Macadamia nuts contain close to
80% monounsaturated fats, the highest of any

fat source, including olive oil. These nuts predominantly contain the beautifying monounsaturated fat called oleic acid *(omega 9)*. They
are the richest source of this beautifying fatty
acid found in any food.

Oleic acid is beneficial in reducing bad cholesterol. It has been shown that the regular
consumption of macadamia nuts protects
against coronary heart disease. Macadamias
nuts, like all other plant foods, contain no significant cholesterol levels.

A diet enriched with oleic acid is associated
with decreased susceptibility of oxidation of
LDL *(bad)* cholesterol and an improvement in
the fluidity of both LDL *(bad)* and HDL *(good)*
cholesterol. An increase in the fluidity of LDL
and HDL decreases arterial clogging.

Although macadamia nuts are high in calories, they contain raw fatty acids that actually
activate the body to more efficiently burn
fats. As a result, less fat accumulates in the
tissues, especially around the heart.

Blood lipid-analysis indicates cholesterol levels on a diet rich in macadamia nuts were similar to a low-fat diet, and lower than the typical
American diet. A macadamia nut diet produces
lower triglyceride levels than other diets.

Macadamia nuts are also the richest natural
source of palmitoleic acid, a monounsaturated fatty acid that acts as an antioxidant, preventing deterioration of cell membranes.
Palmitoleic acid is hydrating and gentle. It
helps to maintain and even restore damaged
or burned skin.

The macadamia nut's overall combination
of oleic fatty acids, palmitoleic fatty acids,
and their significant quantities of zinc makes
these a wonderful skin beautifier.

— How To Select Macadamia Nuts —
While in the shell, choose macadamia nuts
that are large in size and nearly wrinkled on
the outer shell. There will usually only be few
in every batch like this, and they are always
the best tasting.

If purchasing de-shelled nuts, select those that are raw, organic, and whole. If they are split down the middle, or are in pieces, they are usually rancid. Avoid nuts that are overly yellow.

Nettles

Stinging nettles probably originated in Eurasia, although there is some evidence that they were growing in the Americas when the Europeans arrived. Some of the strongest varieties grow in the United Kingdom and Germany.

Mythologically, the Nordics associated nettles with the thunder god Thor. Nettles were perceived to protect one from lightning. The incredible strengthening properties of the nettle plant really do make one more resistal. to the elements.

Nettles are persistent perennials that can grow taller than 2 meters *(6 feet)*. Nettles grow in multiple, thin stalks arising from the ground, somewhat like the hemp plant. Nettle leaves are typically collected, eaten, and/or dried in May and June, just before coming into flower. The stems and leaf-tops of the stinging nettle plant are covered with thin, hair-like protrusions. These protrusions, if touched, release a stinging fluid containing histamine and formic acid. The sting produces a temporary inflammation.

When nettles are eaten, the saliva neutralizes the sting, so that one cannot be stung in the mouth or throat.

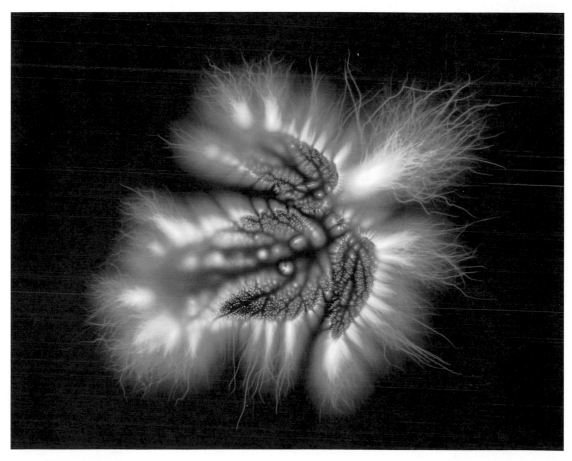

Nettle (*Kirlian Image*)

[the nettle is annoying to the
 _____ poisonous. Ancient shaman
 _____ used to purposely strike their para-
lyzed patients with nettles in order to bring
blood flow back into the muscles and skin.

Nature, in her unique balance, provides the
remedy for the nettle sting by allowing burdock to grow in the same locales as nettles.
Mashed up burdock leaves applied to the
skin relieve nettle stings. Also, the juice from
stinging nettle leaves acts as an antidote to
the sting when topically applied.

Nettle leaves contain a high proportion of
chlorophyll, flavonoids, plant sterols
(immune-system builders), plant enzymes, a
wide range of minerals, and the vitamins A
and C. Nettles contain one of the highest levels of the beautifying mineral silicon found in
any food.

— Weight Loss —

The late wild-food forager, Euell Gibbons,
said that "stinging nettle is very efficacious in
removing unwanted pounds!" Nettle leaves
increase the function of the thyroid gland,
increasing metabolism and helping to burn
away fat while increasing energy. Nettles also
relieve mucus in the colon allowing for the
release of excess waste.

Nettle leaves are so mineral-rich that they
satisfy hunger. This is why it is beneficial to
those with overeating challenges. Overeating
is often an outward manifestation of a search
for minerals. Once the body has the minerals
it is looking for, the desire to eat stops. Eating
food that is fully mineralized eventually
makes us fully mineralized and provides us
with the food-mineral cosmetics necessary to
express true inner and outer beauty.

— Blood Purification Properties —

The nettle, like the burdock root, is best
known as a blood purifier of the highest
caliber. Because of the nettle's high alkaline-
mineral content (silicon and iron) and blood-
building properties, it has earned a reputation
as a beautifier of the highest order.

Nettle leaves are highly alkaline. They neutralize and dissolve acidic wastes in the
blood. Their diuretic properties simultaneously help flush the blood and cleanse it
through the action of the kidneys. Since both
neutralizing and flushing characteristics are
important for blood purification, stinging
nettle is an excellent choice for all complaints
where toxicity and/or over-acidity of the tissues are the root of the problem, including
poor skin quality, weak nails, damaged teeth,
and loss of overall lustre. Its power to purify
the blood will do wonders for chronic skin
ailments. It is effective against eczema on the
upper body, especially of the face, neck, and
ears. This benefit is likely due to its high silicon, chlorophyll, and vitamin C content.

— Nettle Juice —

Gathering nettles and running them
through a juice machine is a unique way to
access the high-quality minerals and oils
present in fresh nettles without having to risk
being stung. This nettle juice is a common
beverage amongst raw-foodists in the United
Kingdom. Every year I do a tour throughout
the United Kingdom, and I always look forward to eating nettles in the English country-
side and drinking nettle juice!

Due to its rich iron content and ease of
absorption, nettle juice is more effective than
spinach juice in building blood.

Given its propensity to neutralize and flush
out acidic waste, nettle juice is perfect for
weight reduction.

Nettle juice can be used as a hair rinse to
restore natural color. Nettle extracts are used
in many shampoos.

— Pharmacology —

Choline acetyltransferase is present in stinging nettle plants, as well as choline, acetyl-
choline, and serotonin. These are all elements of
the nervous system. Serotonin is the most well-
studied neurotransmitter. Although these
elements of the plant have not been studied
in-depth, the presence of these compounds cat-
egorize the nettle as food for the nervous system.

— How To Eat Stinging Nettles —

A friend from England taught me the ancient Druid technique of eating fresh nettles: one comes at the leaf from the bottom, folding it along its central crease, yanking it gently from the mother plant, and then rolling it up so as to enclose the top of the leaf *(where the stingers are most commonly found)*.

For those of us in the real world who want to benefit from nettle nutrition without having to forage in the woods and risk getting stung, a clever way has been devised to make nettles more accessible. This process involves drying the nettles and grinding them into a powder *(thus destroying the stingers)*. This type of powder is used in the superfood, Sun Is Shining. In fact, nettles are the third most prominent ingredient in that blend due to their extraordinary qualities.

Many of us are familiar with nettle tea. It is worth mentioning that the tea is another way to bring the wonderful value of the nettle leaf into your diet. Nettle tea retains many of the beautifying properties of the fresh nettle itself.

Olives and Stone-Crushed Olive Oil

"Olives — their lubricating, cleansing, beautifying, and rejuvenative power is the greatest among all fruits."

— *Vera Richter,*
  The Cook-Less Book

— An Olive Tree —

The olive tree originated in Asia Minor. They may have been under domestication in different regions of the Mediterranean for as long as 10,000 years. The Spanish brought olives to North America and planted them in the Caribbean, and at the missions in California. Today, olive trees are widely cultivated throughout the entire Mediterranean region, and in other locations throughout the world with a similar climate.

Olives come in hundreds of shapes and varieties. They vary widely in taste, even among fruits from the same tree, let alone all the varieties that are currently available.

In classical literature and in the holy writings, olives and olive oil are symbolic of purity, happiness, and abundance.

In Greek mythology, Athena and Poseidon contested over who would become the patron deity of the new city that would eventually become Athens. The pantheon of gods decided that whomever gave the best gift would become patron of the city. Poseidon's

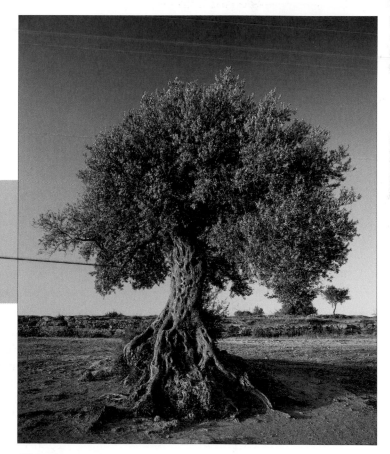

Olive Tree

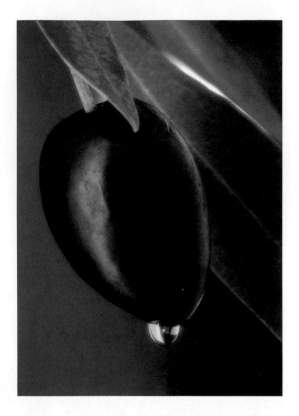

source that is also high in protein *(they have a similar protein-to-fat ratio as red meat)*. Unlike red meat, olives are alkaline, plant-based, and free of chemical injections.

In Arnold Ehret's classic book, *The Mucusless Diet Healing System*, he reprints Ragnar Berg's Table, which organizes different foods by their acid-binding or acid-forming potential. The higher the food's acid-binding potential, the greater its ability to dissolve mucus and cooked-food residues in the body. The olive, it turns out, is the highest mucus dissolver of any fruit. It rates with a value of 30.56, with figs following behind at 27.81. No other fruit in the chart ranks above 20.00. To give you an idea of how high these values are, the orange, an excellent mucus-dissolver, ranks at 9.61.

Olives are high in polyphenols. These are a broad class of water-soluble antioxidants. They display anti-fungal and anti-bacterial properties and are found mostly in the complete olive. However, olive oil does retain a small amount of polyphenols.

An extraordinary beauty-enhancing substance found in olives and olive oil is squalene, which keeps the skin smooth and stimulates the immune system. Chemically, squalene is an unsaturated oil and an oxygen carrier. A related compound called squalane is used in skin care products. Squalane is derived from squalene, but is more stable against oxidation.

Consider the power and benefits of the olive... *(as quoted from The Sunfood Diet Success System):*

1. The highest fruit in minerals.

2. The highest fruit in calcium. Olives contain twice as much calcium as oranges by weight.

3. High in magnesium.

4. High in amino acids, including leucine, aspartic acid, and glutaminic acid.

5. An alkaline fruit.

6. A fatty fruit *(mostly monounsaturated fat)*.

7. An alkaline fat source.

gift was a horse. Athena's gift was the olive tree, which she planted amongst the rocks of the Acropolis in Athens. Due to the superior quality of the olive tree in furthering agriculture, healing, and abundance, Athena won the contest and became the patron goddess of Athens.

Olives played a vital role in Greek culture. The Greek philosopher Thales proved that philosophy was the greatest science, when he predicted that he could, and then successfully did, corner the olive oil market using principles of philosophy.

— Nutrition —

Olives are perhaps the greatest beautifying food of all. Olives and their oil are one of the highest natural sources of vitamin E. This nutrient has been known to erase fine lines on the face, repair connective tissue, heal the circulatory system, and impart its soothing properties upon the digestive tract.

Olives are one of the most perfect body-building foods. They are an alkaline fat

8. Loaded with beneficial omega 3 and omega 6 fatty acids.

9. High in vitamins A and E.

10. In possession of many antioxidant properties. Antioxidants deactivate free radicals, allowing us to live longer, overcome illness, and maintain more acute mental and muscular faculties.

11. Available in different varieties, which fruit throughout the year.

12. Pressable into a powerful oil, usable in a limitless number of ways all year around.

13. Able to soothe the mucous membranes with its oil.

— Green Olives —

Green olives are actually unripe olives, picked early from the tree. At that stage of growth the fruit has not set its full oil and mineral content; therefore, they do not contain as many of the superior nutrients. Freshly-picked green olives are also high in tannic acids, because of this, they are mostly treated with lye *(a harsh alkaline chemical)*.

Only a few varieties of green olives exist that are not treated with lye. These are available several months of the year.

— How To Select Olives —

Olives, as they naturally ripen under a tree, are perishable. They ripen irregularly. In their natural state, one really has to know how to select properly ripened olives. They are difficult to harvest and distribute in their natural state. However, this can be done. Sunfood Nutrition's Peruvian Olives are done this way. These olives are naturally ripened and remain free of any kind of treatment.

In most cases, however, to be able to uniformly distribute olives and ensure quality, olives are typically either water-cured, salted, and/or altered in some other way. The best way to adjust the ripening process is to water cure or sun-dry the olives in salty water.

Vinegar-pickled olives are fine; they are acid forming in the digestive process, even though technically not cooked. This may actually be beneficial to some as the vinegar acids assist the stomach acids in the digestion of food.

Canned black olives have been pasteurized *(cooked)* and soaked in ferrous gluconate *(an iron compound that darkens them)* and should be avoided. The only cured olives I recommend eating are either done with vinegar, or they are "water-cured" or "sea-salted."

— How To Use Olives —
Olives greatly enhance salads and raw-food cuisine of all types. They also make great snack foods and party appetizers with vegetables.

Olive Oil

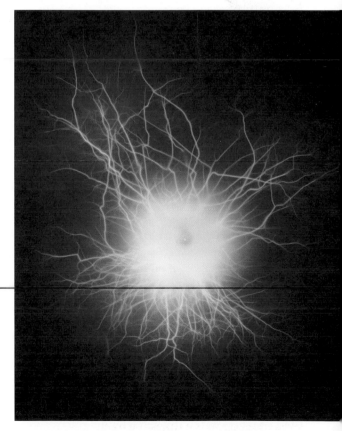

A Drop of Stone-Crushed Olive Oil (*Kirlian Image*)

Olive oil lubricated the machines of the Roman Empire all the way into the industrial revolution. Olive oil illuminated Mediterranean homes well into the 19th century.

Hippocrates, the most famous Greek physician of ancient times, recommended olive oil for healing ulcers, cholera, and muscular pains. In more recent medical times, the health and beautifying benefits of olive oil have received considerable attention.

— Fatty-Acid Content —
The primary fatty acids in olive oil are oleic, linoleic and linolenic acid. Oleic acid is a beautifying monounsaturated fat and makes up 55-85% of the oil. Linoleic is polyunsaturated and makes up approximately 9%. Linolenic, which is polyunsaturated, makes up 0.0-1.5% of the oil.

— Olive Oil —
Lowers Heart Disease Risks
Many widely-published studies reveal that the consumption of olive oil by Mediterranean peoples is a major reason why they have a far lower incidence of heart disease than Americans.

Investigators at Harvard conducted a survey of Greek women to determine if their abundant consumption of olive oil could also increase cancer risk. Their findings indicated that olive oil had an opposite effect. They concluded that the breast cancer risk for women who consume olive oil more than once per day is reduced by 25 percent when compared to women who consume olive oil less frequently. "Our work shows an association between consumption of a type of fat and reduced risk of breast cancer," said Dr. Dimitrios Trichopoulos, director of the study. "These findings suggest that the type of fat source one consumes may influence breast cancer risk in opposite directions."

— Cooking —
For cooking purposes, olive oil is better than polyunsaturated vegetable oils (corn oil, canola oil, safflower oil, etc.) and margarine. It is, however, still susceptible to heat-caused oxidation that changes the chemical structure

of the oil into harmful trans-fatty acids. The best choice for a cooking oil is coconut oil.

— How To Use Olive Oil —
Olive oil greatly enhances salads of all types. It is also a great addition to fruit smoothies because it slows down the absorption of fruit sugars so that the energy one derives from the smoothie is longer lasting. In the Mediterranean, people still have two tablespoons of olive oil as their first food for breakfast each morning.

— Skin and Olive Oil —
Olive oil is a soothing fat for damaged and dry skin, hair, and nails. It can be used to soothe the skin after shaving. It also may be used on baby skin. To moisturize dry skin and heal skin damage, one may apply olive oil daily and directly to dry spots and stretch marks.

The ancient Greeks used to bathe with olive oil, using a special scraper to take off the excess.

After a hot evening bath or shower, massaging olive oil into the skin makes a great before-bed treatment. Allow the oil to soak in for twenty minutes and towel off any excess.

— How To Select Olive Oil —
Stone-crushed olive oil is made from olives crushed and ground with stone presses using the original techniques developed thousands of years ago by the Greeks and Romans. Olive oil should be organic, extra-virgin, stone-crushed, cold-pressed, and stored in dark glass bottles (oils are light sensitive).

The difference between virgin and extra-virgin olive oils is their acidity level, which affects their taste and quality. Extra-virgin varieties have fewer acids.

— Dark Glass Bottles —
Olive oil should be packaged in dark glass bottles. Researchers have shown that olive oil stored in polyethylene bottles exposed to light can develop unacceptable amounts of damaging peroxides in as little as twenty days. If stored in dark bottles the oil can last at least 120-190 days, and evidence suggests

that stone-crushed olive oil packaged in dark bottles can last as long as two years.

Oil deteriorates through the action of oxygen and the enzyme lipase found in the oil. Oxidation or rancidity speeds up with light and heat exposure. It is best to keep olive oil in a cool, dark cabinet. It can also be put into the refrigerator or freezer without much harm; this will extend its shelf life. However, constantly warming and then rechilling olive oil *(causing it to go from a solid to liquid and back again)* will corrode the olive oil more quickly — and this will negatively affect its taste.

— Stone-Crushed Olive Oil —

Most olive oils are pressed in giant machines that reach destructive temperatures above 160 degrees Fahrenheit, even though they are claimed to be "cold-pressed." They are also typically highly refined and filtered, and contain very little, if any, minerals.

The Romans were the first to perfect the stone press with which they extracted the olive's oil. Stone-crushed olive oil retains richer tastes, more minerals, and purer nutrients. One simple taste is enough to convince anyone of the superiority of stone-crushed olive oil. It must be stone-crushed and cold-pressed to maintain the quality of minerals and nutrients necessary to experience its health- and skin-enhancing qualities.

Onions

Some archaeologists, botanists, and food historians believe onions originated in central Asia, Iran, and/or West Pakistan, but nobody is quite sure because onions were found growing in the Americas when the Pilgrims arrived.

It is likely that our ancestors ate wild onions long before the beginning of agriculture. This simple vegetable was probably a major staple in the prehistoric diet. Research indicates that they have been cultivated for at least 5,000 years, and probably much longer. They may have been simultaneously domesticated in different regions. Onions were probably one of the first domesticated crops because they

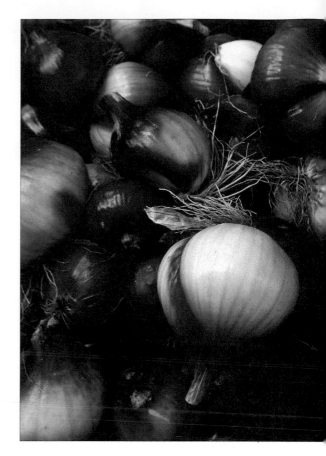

are easy to grow, easy to transport, and have a long life after picking.

There are many ancient documents that describe the use of onions in art, medicine, and mummification.

Over 5,000 years ago, onions grew in the earliest Chinese gardens. They are mentioned in the Vedic writings from India. In Egypt, onions were in use over 5,000 years ago. There are tablets confirming that the Sumerians were growing them over 4,500 years ago. Onions are also mentioned in the Bible *(Numbers 11:5)*.

To the Egyptians, the onion bulb was worshipped as a symbol of the universe. It was considered a sacred symbol of the mother-goddess, Isis. The layer-upon-layer structure of the onion symbolized eternity to the Egyptians, who buried onions along with their Pharaohs. In the tombs and in some of the pyramids of Egypt, onions are pictured in the hands of priests. They are shown covering altars and they are depicted on feasting banquet tables. Often Egyptian workers were paid in onions.

Dioscorides, a Greek physician who lived 2,000 years ago, noted several medicinal uses for onions. The Greeks employed onions to strengthen athletes for the Olympic Games. Before their sporting matches, Olympic athletes would eat onions, drink onion juice, and rub onions on their bodies.

The Romans ate onions and carried them on journeys to provinces throughout the empire. The Roman scholar Pliny the Elder described that onions can disinfect dog bites, heal mouth sores and poor vision, induce sleep, and alleviate toothaches and dysentery.

By the Middle Ages in Europe, onions had become one of the major staple vegetables. They were prescribed to alleviate burns, flesh wounds, hair loss, headaches, parasites, snakebites, and upset stomachs. Onions were applied to the skin to quickly heal bruises — a remedy that is still used today. They were also used as rent payments and wedding gifts.

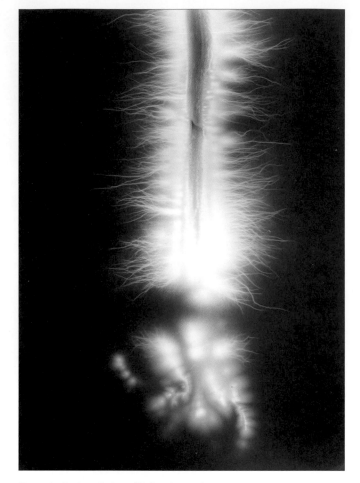

Organic Spring Onion *(Kirlian Image)*

— Sulfur Content of Onions —

Sulfur, as we have seen, is a beautifier of the highest order because it cleanses the liver and skin, has antiseptic properties, and helps to build all connective tissue.

The onion contains a considerable amount of sulfuric oils, which stimulate the mucus lining of the sinuses and digestive organs. Cutting up onions, as we know, can bring one to tears. Internally, these stimulating oils increase the flow of digestive juices creating a greater absorption of nutrients.

The sulfuric oils in onions have antiseptic qualities. They prevent putrefaction in the intestines and inhibit the growth of harmful bacteria in the digestive tract. These oils help alleviate coughs, sore throats, and congested lungs and sinuses.

Mixed with honey *(which tones down the sulfuric compounds)*, onion juice is good for hoarseness and coughs. Externally, this honey/onion juice mix can be applied to infected wounds to aid healing.

Onions combine wonderfully with avocados, nuts, seeds of all different types, and almost any other type of fat or oil because fats and oils tone down the sulfuric compounds. When onions are eaten with a fat or oil, each makes the other more digestible.

— Quercetin —

Onions contain the anti-cancer, anti-microbial phytochemicals known as disulfides, trisulfides, cepaene, and vinyl dithiins — yet the most unique compound in onions is quercetin.

Studies have indicated that onions are the highest source of usable quercetin *(an antioxidant flavonoid)*, surpassing other good sources such as apples and tea. Quercetin helps to eliminate free radicals in the body to protect and regenerate the beauty vitamin *(vitamin E)*, to inactivate the harmful effects of heavy metals, and to decrease capillary fragility *(a useful factor in healing varicose veins)*.

Foods from the allium family, which includes onions, chives, leeks, and of course garlic, are all good for alleviating varicose veins. They help to keep the veins and capillaries elastic and flexible.

Several studies have shown quercetin to have unique beneficial effects against many disorders, including cataracts and cardiovascular disease, as well as with breast, colon, ovarian, gastric, lung, and bladder cancers.

— Blood Clumping — (Platelet Aggregation)

University of Wisconsin-Madison researchers found that onions exhibit strong anti-blood clumping activity. Onions cause thick, clumped blood to thin out. Blood clumping is a term for the stickiness of red-blood cells in the blood stream; this is sometimes called platelet aggregation. Blood clumping is associated with atherosclerosis, cardiovascular disease, heart attacks, impotency, and strokes.

Because onions thin the blood by dispersing fat and protein, they allow for the uptake of more oxygen while decreasing the possibility of heart disease. More oxygen in the blood stream brings more richness to the complexion.

— Longevity —

My friend and world-renowned food-researcher, Dr. John Heinerman, in his book, *Heinerman's Encyclopedia of Herbs and Spices*, details the research of the late Belle Boone Beard, a sociologist who once worked for the National Institute of Aging. During her career, Beard had interviewed over 8,500 centenarians *(people who live to 100 and beyond)*. One thing she noticed was the commonality of onions in the diet of those she interviewed. Nearly everyone who reached 100+ years enjoyed eating onions. Some declared that they ate onions with every meal, every day! Beard came to believe that onions played a major role in longevity.

— Other Properties —

Onions resist hybridization and are capable of reverting back to the wild state more readily than almost any other food. This means that onions have a strong vital life force that they impart upon the consumer. They are able to uptake and create minerals as well as, or better than, nearly any other food, making them a fantastic mineralizer.

A typical onion contains more vitamin C than an orange of the same size. Onions also contain vitamin A, thiamin, niacin, riboflavin, folic acid, sulfur *(as we have noted)*, calcium, phosphorus, potassium, iron, silicon, fiber, and a high protein quality *(this means they have a high ratio of milligrams of amino acids to grams of protein)*.

Author and lecturer, Dr. David Jubb, believes that onions increase the strength of orgasms due to their ability to cleanse and prepare for a parasympathetic flush of the lymphatic system.

Select onions that are hard, juicy, and free from mold. I like to eat all kinds of onions depending on my mood. For fancy dinners I choose red onions. If I am enjoying lots of rich nuts in my salad, I like strong white onions. Yellow onions are not as strong as white. Due to their mild nature, green onions go well with a lunch-time meal.

Papaya

The papaya originated on the lowlands above the geographical limestone shelves of eastern Central America, where it still grows wild today. In the 1500s, Spanish and Portuguese sailors took to the fruit and spread it to their other settlements in the West and East Indies. The papaya was then taken to the tropical Pacific Islands. Eventually, the papaya reached all tropical regions. Hardier varieties even grow in some subtropical locales.

Papaya trees may grow to be 10 meters *(30 feet)* tall. They look somewhat like palms with their characteristic branchless tree trunk shaft. Atop this shaft rests a radiating crest of giant uniquely-cut leaves, beneath which a cluster of fruits is typically found. The large ovoid fruit grows like a melon and can range in size from 0.5 to 9 kilograms *(1 to 20 pounds)*.

The papaya tree is an amazingly generous producer of fruit. In mineral-rich tropical regions, papayas can grow from a seed to a fruiting, seed-bearing plant in 9 months!

Varying widely in size, shape, and color, the most common varieties of papaya are yellow, orange, or red-skinned. Hawaiian papayas are a bit smaller than other varieties.

The Hawaiian fruits are fist-sized and pack a strawberry-like flavor. Mexican papayas grow much larger. One Mexican variety I often purchase in Tijuana is the rosa "red" papaya, which has a high enzyme content.

The sweet flesh of the papaya is melon-like, yet softer. In the center of the fruit rest edible, yet very spicy, black peppercorn-like seeds.

In their flesh, papayas contain a large quantity of alkaline minerals *(especially calcium)*, vitamin A *(unusual for a fruit)*, and a high concentration of collagen-healing vitamin C.

Papayas cleanse and soothe the digestive tract. They help calm indigestion, and alleviate flatulence. After eating two medium-sized papayas each day for a week, one will feel remarkably cleansed from the inside out. Papayas greatly enhance skin beauty, nail strength, and hair lustre. Raw-foodists who eat papaya regularly develop radiant, glowing eyes.

In many countries, especially Mexico, papaya juice is a favorite delicacy. The juice can be applied topically to lighten freckles and nourish the skin. As a food, it makes for a tasty, cleansing, nourishing beverage that retains all the properties of the fruit flesh.

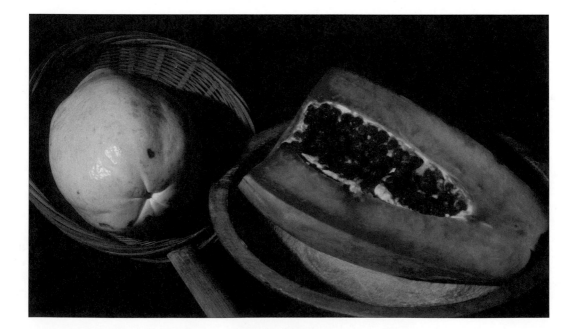

— Papain —

Unripe to three-quarters-ripe papayas contain a high concentration of a unique protease enzyme called papain. Protease is a protein-splitting enzyme similar to the stomach enzyme pepsin. Papain is renowned for its anti-cancer and skin cleansing properties. The enzyme is present in the fresh milky juice of the unripe fruit, and in the brownish powder that remains after the milky juice dries. Very little of this enzyme is found in the fully ripe fruit.

Due to their remarkable skin-enhancing qualities, papaya enzymes have come into vogue in the cosmetic skin-care industry. Remember, the skin is nourished by a diet rich in enzymes *(from raw-foods)* and minerals. When half-ripe papayas are both eaten and applied to the skin, their enzymes soften and dissolve dead skin layers, while simultaneously the alkaline minerals nourish and support the creation of healthy skin. The enzymes immediately set to work tightening the skin's collagen tissue. Enzymes are capable of protecting and repairing elastic collagen fibers, which both protect us against wrinkles and alleviate existing skin damage.

— Papaya Facial Treatment —

To cleanse and clarify the skin, obtain three-quarters-ripe papayas, cut the fruit, and rub your face with the fruit. The more unripe the fruit, the stronger the enzymes will be. Beware: if the enzymes are too strong, they can burn the skin, particularly the delicate membranes around the eyes and lips. Let the fruit soak in for 5-10 minutes, before washing. After a treatment with papaya, the complexion appears youthful, radiant, and fresh.

— Papaya Healing Properties —

Papain has anti-cancer properties, as the enzymes eat the protein-laden material surrounding certain cancerous tumors. Half-ripe papayas are typically prescribed by raw-food nutritionists for women with breast cancer. This is because the enzyme content is higher, and the sugar content of the fruit is lower *(low-sugar diets are generally recommended for cancer)*.

Recent research demonstrates that eating papayas reduces the risk of arteriosclerosis, strokes, and heart attacks. This is partially due to carpaine, an alkaloid compound in papayas with anti-tumor properties and organ-healing qualities. Carpaine lowers the concentration of fats and cholesterol in the blood stream. It also helps to regenerate a hardened, dysfunctional liver.

— Anti-Parasite Properties —

The black peppercorn seeds inside the papaya may be eaten. They have a sulfur-rich peppery taste, much like wild mustard, arugula, and watercress. One tablespoon of seeds chewed up each day can both guard against, and flush out, parasites. This is especially important to know if one is *(or has been)* traveling or living in the tropics.

Papaya seeds can be used either fresh or dried. For maximum effectiveness, one tablespoon of fresh seeds should be chewed well and eaten once a day on an empty stomach. If the taste of plain seeds is too strong, mix with dates or honey. Dried or fresh seeds may also be blended into drinking water. As an anti-parasite program, consume papaya seeds once a day for a week, and then repeat the treatment two weeks later. If traveling in parasite-friendly tropical regions, papaya seeds should be eaten every day.

— How To Eat Papayas —

To eat a papaya, slice the fruit in half *(lengthwise)* and scoop out the seeds and juicy flesh. Discard the skin. Papaya combines wonderfully with sliced avocados for breakfast. Papaya juice is also a welcome alternative to orange juice in the morning.

The spicy black seeds are crunchy. They can be used as a garnish, as a substitute for capers, or blended into a salad dressing to add spice.

— How To Select Papayas —

I usually get my papayas from a friendly fruit seller in Tijuana, just over the border from my home town of San Diego, California. Tijuana has an incredible fruit market *(fruiteria)*. I often go with friends and family to drink fresh coconuts and buy exotic fruits not available in the United States.

When I look for ready-to-eat papayas, I look for those with deep red, orange, or dark yellow skins *(depending on the variety)*. The more green on the papaya, the more unripe. I select papayas that possess a gentle softness in the skin. I avoid overly soft or bruised fruit, or any with soft or hard spots. I also choose fruits that feel heavy for their size.

Pumpkin Seeds

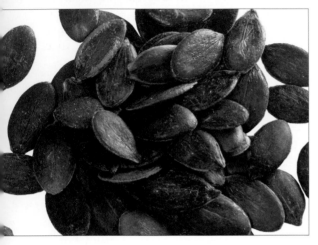

References to pumpkins date back far into the recesses of time. The name "pumpkin" originated from the Greek word "pepon," which means a "large, sun-ripened melon." Pepon was passed into the French language as the word "pompon." The English changed "pompon" to "pumpion." American colonists changed "pumpion" into "pumpkin." They became popularized through such folk tales as *The Legend of Sleepy Hollow, Peter The Pumpkin Eater*, and *Cinderella*. Pumpkins have always been present in North America, where they have been a staple winter food of the natives.

Pumpkins are part of the cucumber/melon family, which includes gourds, melons, and squash. All pumpkin and squash seeds are edible. Most varieties produce seeds that are enclosed in ovoid-shaped shells thin enough

to crack open with your teeth. Some pumpkin varieties have shell-less seeds and are grown specifically because they are easy to eat. In the early 1970s, the U.S. Department of Agriculture bred a new, high-yield pumpkin cultivar called Lady Godiva, containing rounded, dark green, shell-less seeds. This variety is seen in many health-food stores today.

Pumpkin seeds are a wonderful source of B vitamins, many minerals *(including zinc)*, phytonutrients *(cucurbitin phytosterol)*, and essential fatty oils. They contain hormone-building elements. The oils in these seeds not only support normal sexual function but also help protect against heart disease. They have traditionally been used for prostate disorders. They supply a safe and natural source of tryptophan *(the least abundant amino acid in most people's diets)*. These seeds help remove intestinal worms. They contain myosin, the chief protein constituent of nearly all muscles in the body, which strengthens muscle contraction. The seeds also contain vitamin B17, otherwise known as laetrile or amygdalin *(which has reputed anti-tumor and anti-cancer effects)*.

— Fatty Acids —

Pumpkin seeds are an excellent source of unsaturated fatty acids, including oleic fatty acids, as well as omega 3 and omega 6 essential fatty acids. Oleic acid has strong beautifying properties *(similar to macadamia nuts)*. The anti-inflammatory, antioxidant omega 3 fatty acids produce clear, radiant skin and protect from ultra-violet radiation.

Pumpkin-seed oil has been used throughout history in India, Europe, and the Americas. This dark green, flavor-rich oil should be cold-pressed and kept in dark containers. It can be used in raw-food recipes and on salads. It contains a nice proportion of omega 3 and omega 6 essential fatty acids. The seed oil is helpful for healing burns and wounds.

— Zinc —

As we have seen, zinc improves the ability to smell and taste. It activates hundreds of enzyme systems *(especially those involved with connective tissue and digestion).* Warts, acne, and skin conditions are improved significantly when one consumes more zinc-rich foods.

Pumpkin seeds are nature's most perfect food for the prostate gland due to their high magnesium and zinc content. Chronic prostate inflammation is linked to a lack of dietary zinc. Researchers have found that sunflower and pumpkin seeds have a positive effect on symptoms for both BPH *(benign prostatic hypertrophy)* and prostatitis. In Germany, nettle root *(Urtica dioica)* and pumpkin seeds *(Cucurbita pepo)* are also approved for treatment of BPH *(Fortschritte der Medizin, 1996, vol. 10).* A clinical, placebo-controlled study found that pumpkin seeds in combination with saw palmetto significantly improved BPH without side effects *(British Journal of Urology, 1990, vol. 66).*

Pumpkin seeds are a true aphrodisiac because, in men, they pump the prostate full of zinc, build seminal fluid, and increase sperm count. In women, they build hormones, activate the sexual organs, and increase sexual fluid secretions.

— Tryptophan —

Raw pumpkin seeds are one of the best sources of the amino acid tryptophan. This amino acid is one of the least common in most people's diets because tryptophan is intolerant to high-heat and is destroyed by cooking.

Tryptophan works with tyrosine and zinc to improve one's mood and increase levels of serotonin in the brain, alleviating depression and brain chemistry imbalances caused by using drugs such as MDMA *(Ecstasy).* Anecdotal reports relate that pumpkin seeds and durian *(another good source of tryptophan)* create a mild euphoria and relieve stress. Tryptophan's relaxing qualities help to alleviate insomnia.

— Anti-Parasite Effect —

Pumpkin seeds may be taken as a safe de-worming agent. They are particularly useful against tapeworms in children and pregnant women, when stronger, harsher herbs are inappropriate.

To use pumpkin seeds to rid the body of intestinal parasites *(tapeworms or roundworms),* eat a handful of raw seeds twice a day on an empty stomach for one week. Take a week off, and then repeat this process again for another week. If eaten with garlic, pumpkin seeds are even effective in flushing out pinworms.

Researchers have isolated an amino acid called cucurbitin, found primarily in pumpkin seeds and certain related species, that is likely responsible for the worm-expelling effects. Cucurbitin is believed to paralyze worms, causing them to loosen their grip, and then allowing them to be expelled from the body.

There are no known side effects or reports of toxicity regarding pumpkin seeds.

— How To Prepare Pumpkin Seeds —

Many times I simply eat pumpkin seeds in their natural state. Sometimes I soak them in water for half a day and then dehydrate them in the sun or in a dehydrator. Soaking nuts or seeds in water removes the enzyme inhibitors, allowing for easier digestion. Enzyme inhibitors are present in unsprouted nuts and seeds in order to keep them in a dormant state until the ideal conditions are present for their sprouting.

— How To Select Pumpkin Seeds —

Pumpkin seeds vary in size and shape. Some are tan in color, others are dark green. I select organic seeds that are crisp, rather than flimsy and pliable. In Mexico, pumpkin seeds are sometimes called pepitas, and may also be labeled as such in North America.

Raw pumpkin-seed butter *(made of ground-down pumpkin seeds)* is available in some health-food stores and through mail order.

Radishes

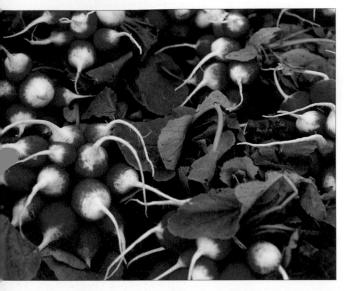

Radishes are a dominant member of the mustard family. They were originally cultivated in central Asia or China. They grow wildly all over Europe and the Mediterranean. The Europeans likely introduced them to the Americas, where they now grow wildly.

Herodotus wrote in *History (II, cxxv)* that the builders of the Great Pyramid were fed radishes, onions, and garlic.

Radishes are perhaps the most beautifying of all foods. The radishes' rejuvenative properties are found in their high sulfur, silicon, and vitamin C content. Radishes are the only common food with both sulfur and silica found in high concentrations. Radishes are

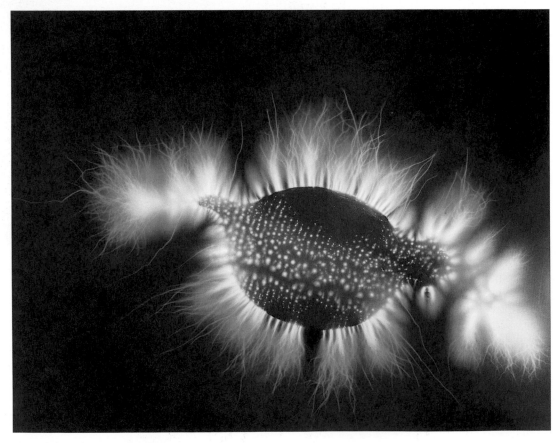

Organic Radish (*Kirlian Image*)

one of the highest vegetable sources of vitamin C, which plays a major role in connective tissue formation. Both of the minerals *(silicon and sulfur)* work together with vitamin C to create glowing skin.

Red radishes seem to be the most beautifying because of their high silicon content. Daikon radishes are also excellent, but not as strong. Black radishes are very powerful mucus-dissolvers, and are high in sulfur.

Black radishes are Professor Arnold Ehret's #1 mucus-dissolving food *(as mentioned in his book, The Mucusless Diet Healing System).*

Radishes are effective at cutting and dissolving mucus in the digestive tract — especially the mucus formed from eating starchy carbohydrates such as bread, pasta, and rice. They stimulate the liver, relax bile ducts, increase bile flow, help cleanse the system, expel and prevent gallstones, and, as an overall result, increase the digestive fires.

The sulfurous mustard oil in radishes stimulates the circulatory system, contributing to skin radiance.

Radishes are used in Russia for both hypothyroidism and hyperthyroidism. Raphanin, a substance in radishes, helps keep levels of thyroid hormones in balance, allowing one to remain at their perfect weight.

Radishes also contain quite a bit of folic acid *(vitamin B9)*, making them great nerve strengtheners.

Radishes are great kidney cleansers and thus decrease water retention and improve elimination. Radish juice is effective in helping to alleviate the pain caused by kidney stones; this juice even helps dissolve kidney stones.

— How To Eat Radishes —

Little red radishes make an excellent snack food. They can also be tossed into salads and added to fresh vegetable juices.

Radishes can also be sliced thin, soaked in a small amount of olive oil, sea salt, and spices and then dehydrated to make savory snacks.

— How To Select Radishes —

Select radishes that are fresh and crisp to the bite. If they become flimsy, they are old.

Black radishes are generally in season from the winter through the spring. Other radishes may be found in stores during all seasons.

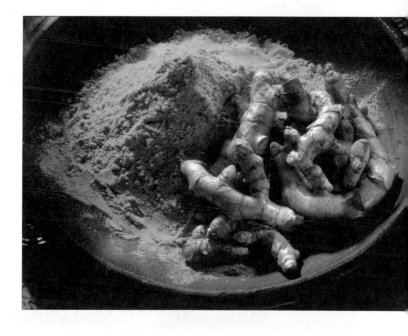

Turmeric

Turmeric probably originated in tropical parts of India and most likely was first domesticated there.

Turmeric is a root and member of the ginger family. It has a similar shape and consistency to ginger. It is best known in its yellow powdered form, which is commonly used as a spicy and warming food/herb in India.

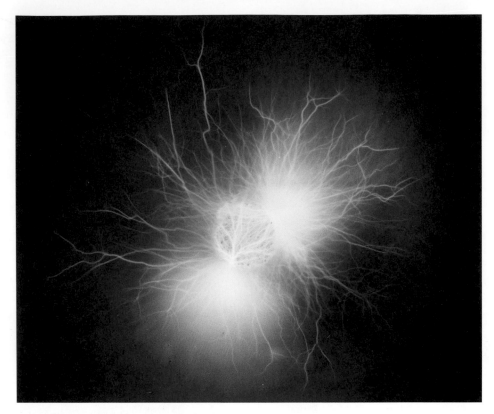

Slice of Organic Turmeric *(Kirlian Image)*

Turmeric is widely used in Ayurvedic medicine for its beautifying properties and is well-renowned as nature's internal cosmetic.

Generally considered a restorative food, turmeric displays strong anti-inflammatory, antioxidant, anti-cancer, and anti-microbial characteristics.

— Antioxidant Properties —
Curcumin, a flavonoid within turmeric, is the antioxidant substance responsible for its anti-cancer and anti-inflammatory effects. In tests, curcumin's anti-inflammatory effects were found to be on par with the drugs cortisone and phenylbutazone.

— Blood Purification —
Turmeric is a first-class blood purifier. It stimulates the liver, increases red-blood cell formation, inhibits red-blood-cell clumping, and increases circulation. This allows wounds to heal faster and exhausted tissues to rejuvenate. Clean blood corrects both excesses and deficiencies in metabolism and increases one's energy.

— Skin —
Turmeric makes the skin soft, supple, and smooth. Beautiful skin results from pure blood. Because turmeric helps to purify the blood, it helps to counteract pimples, acne, boils, and similar skin imbalances.

Turmeric brings color into pale skin. It adds juiciness to dry skin. It affects the complexion as profoundly as any food. In the art of radiant beauty, these kinds of results are a sure sign that food really does affect us.

— How To Select Turmeric —
Fresh turmeric root should resemble ginger, only smaller, orange, and more profusely branching. Turmeric powder is bright yellow and has a slightly spicy taste when unadulterated.

— How To Use Turmeric —

Turmeric can be used in place of ginger. It may be added to salad dressings, smoothies, and various raw-food recipes.

A small 2.5 centimeter (1 inch) piece of turmeric put through a juice machine will spice up a quart of fresh juice.

Another turmeric drink can be made by mixing 1-2 teaspoons of turmeric powder into a smoothie. This can be drunk once or twice a day.

Turmeric oil may be applied externally as a beautifier. To create an external application of turmeric oil, mix 30 grams (1 ounce) of powdered turmeric in a 1/2 liter (pint) of sesame oil. Allow this mixture to steep in a warm place for two weeks, and then strain out the residue through a cloth.

An old folk remedy for canker sores is turmeric and honey. At the earliest sign of a canker sore, make a paste with 1 tablespoon of honey and 1/4 tablespoon of powdered turmeric. Apply this directly to the sore. The honey acts as a sealant to keep in the antiseptic elements of the turmeric.

Watercress

Watercress is a common green-leafy vegetable that grows in riparian areas (near natural springs, small creeks, and streams). Its origins are unclear, as it grows abundantly throughout the northern hemisphere.

An old legend says that when watercress is eaten at the day's end it increases dreams that evening. This is probably due to its high concentration of minerals.

Watercress contains a complex array of minerals and trace minerals that help heal anemia, endocrine imbalances (including thyroid and pituitary deficiencies), osteoporosis, and a host of mineral-deficient conditions. It has an affinity for the skin and is effective in helping to heal chronic cases of eczema, pimples, acne, etc.

Watercress and arugula share many similar qualities. They taste similar and are both cruciferous vegetables in the mustard family. Yet, watercress contains significantly higher amounts of beautifying micronutrients, such as sulfur, manganese, iodine, iron, copper, calcium, and vitamins A, B1, B2, C, and E. It contains three times as much vitamin E as lettuce and three times as much calcium as spinach. Iodine, a thyroid mineral, is rarely found in land-based plants.

Watercress, like arugula, is highly alkaline. It neutralizes acidic waste products throughout the blood and lymphatic system. It increases circulation while simultaneously delivering minerals to the cells. This brings color and lustre into the skin, face, lips, eyes, and hair.

Watercress contains mustard glycosides and mustard oil, which are internal antiseptics and internal tissue and skin cleansers.

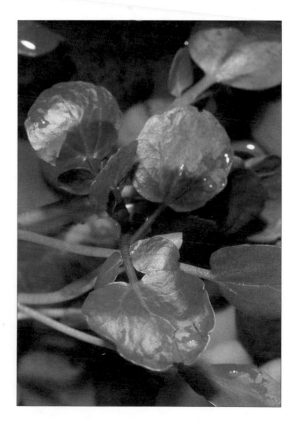

— How To Select Watercress —

When selecting watercress in the store, look for strong, vigorous, fresh-picked bunches. Avoid weak or wilted leaves.

Watercress tastes best when picked before the plant flowers and goes to seed. To harvest watercress, simply pick the young leaves and the plant will keep regrowing new ones for months.

— How To Eat Watercress —

Watercress makes an excellent addition to any salad. Mixing it in a salad with avocados and olive oil tends to calm the leaves' spicy elements and makes this food more digestible.

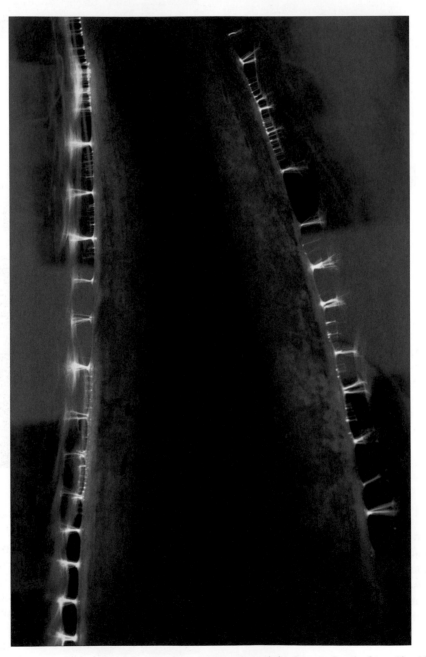

Aloe Vera *(Kirlian Image)* — we have now reviewed the Beauty Foods from Aloe Vera to Watercress. Of course, this listing of Beauty Foods is only a beginning.

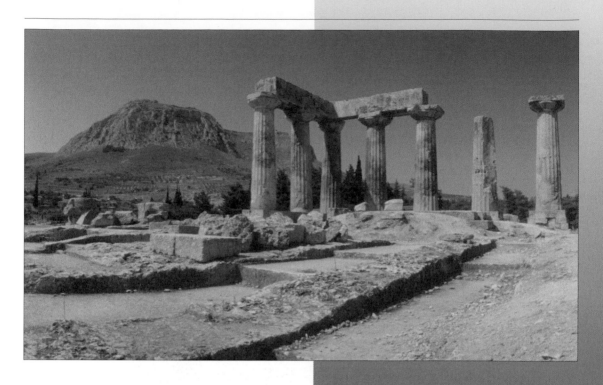

The Beauty Diet® is based on the laws of beauty, which allow you to create habits of beauty that manifest themselves physically as patterns of beauty.

Beauty is found in flowing form, grace, electromagnetism, and symmetry. These are the admirable culinary qualities that make raw-foods so wonderful.

Adopting the raw-food lifestyle will put you in nature's beauty parlor. It will bring color and vibrancy back into your complexion and cuisine. The Beauty Diet® erases fine lines and creates moisture and smoothness in the skin.

The benefits of The Beauty Diet® are often subtle and increase in intensity as you develop more habits of beauty. There is never something for nothing in this world. "Anything worth having is worth working for" was Andrew Carnegie's insightful and truthful saying. Things of true value are only attained through a test of faith.

If your choice is to move into totally embracing the raw-food approach, I recom-mend that in addition to studying this book, you read my book *The Sunfood Diet Success System* and some recipe companions includ-ing *Raw Transformation* and *Rawvolution*. I also recommend that, instead of taking haphazard advice from any of the common diet books, you visit with your local healthcare practi-tioner and have yourself tested for food aller-gies. Any foods that you are allergic to should be avoided. Allergic reactions will cause inflammation and decrease beauty.

If any of the advice in this lesson is outside your understanding or ability to use right now, skip over it. The essence of eating raw-plant-food is to simplify. Make the process simple and fun!

Key Reminders
— Chlorophyll —
In designing a diet suitable for you, be sure to consider the alkalizing, healing, and nourishing effects of green, chlorophyll-rich foods.

There is no healer quite like chlorophyll. Eat at least one green salad each day — two if you can. Drink one or two 12-ounce glasses of a green drink each day (a fresh vegetable juice and/or a drink containing 1-3 tablespoons of a green superfood powder, such as Sun Is Shining or Pure Synergy).

— Water —
Remember to drink water at least 30 minutes before meals, instead of during or after meals.

— Food Combining —
As a general rule, start out each day with lighter foods and move toward heavier foods later in the day. Heavy foods for breakfast can weigh an individual down throughout the day.

A rule of transition is to make eating cooked meals more simple. Eat only one type of cooked food or animal food at each meal, and always have raw salad vegetables and salad fruits (tomatoes, cucumbers, bell peppers, etc.) with it.

— Alcohol —
If you enjoy alcohol with dinner, consider a healthy choice, such as an organic, sulfite-free wine. Numerous studies have now demonstrated that wine, when consumed in moderate amounts, provides antioxidant (flavonol and resveratrol) protection against numerous cardiovascular problems. However, if one really wants even healthier cardiovascular support, dark chocolate — especially raw chocolate (cacao beans or cacao nibs, which are raw pieces of the chocolate nut) contain even more cardiovascular supporting antioxidants than wine. Please see my book Naked Chocolate for more details on the true power of chocolate. For the best high-end chocolate bars ever, please search Sacred Chocolate at www.sunfood.com.

— Daily Menus —
The following menus are suggestions only. They provide an idea of what to eat every day. They are not rules, only tools to help raw-food nutrition become part of your beauty program. You can use these menus to guide you towards a 100% raw-diet. Other than MSM and chaparral tea, all supplement ideas are included in the next section.

BREAKFAST IDEAS

Daily Essentials
- 1/2 liter (quart) of water mixed with 1/2 tablespoon of MSM crystals.

Raw Choices
- Any of the following types of fresh fruit: papaya, figs, grapes, berries, melons, apples, grapefruits, pineapple, etc.
- A smoothie containing superfoods (see Lesson 10: Beauty Recipes under Smoothies for ideas).
- A fruit salad (see Lesson 10: Beauty Recipes under Papaya Salad for ideas).

Heated or Cooked Choices
- 1/4 liter (8 ounces) of herbal tea. Squeeze in fresh lemon if desired. Use fresh maple syrup or raw honey to sweeten.
- Oatmeal (Steel-cut oats are best. Oats contain the beauty mineral silicon).
- Toast with coconut butter/oil or 1/2 avocado (made from whole grain bread or sprouted bread). Toast is easier to digest than regular bread.

LUNCH IDEAS

Raw Choices
- 1 shot *(1-2 fluid ounces)* of wheatgrass juice. *(Wheatgrass tends to suppress the appetite.)*
- 1 liter *(quart)* of fresh vegetable juice containing at least 50% green vegetables, 50% apples or pears.
- One small leafy-green vegetable salad. *(see Lesson 10: Beauty Recipes under Salads for ideas.)*
- Guacamole *(avocado, cilantro, olives, lime juice, tomatoes, onions, celtic sea salt, etc.)*.
- One durian *(fresh, if possible...frozen is okay, if fresh cannot be found)*. One whole durian is a big meal!
- Cantaloupe *(contains a high amount of beta-carotene and antioxidants)*.

Heated or Cooked Choices
- One sandwich containing toasted sprouted grain bread, avocado, clover and radish sprouts, diced red bell pepper, sliced olives, onion, and diced cucumber.
- Rice *(or bean)* burrito containing lettuce, onions, lime juice, and tomatoes. No cheese.

Animal-Based Foods
(Including animal-based foods in one's diet is an individual choice. I do not include them in my diet. Fish and wild game are more mineral-rich, contain better quality oils, and leaner protein. Goat's milk is much more digestible than cow's milk. Most of the world's population is allergic to cow's milk).
- Smoked fish *(only from clean, organic sources — not herring, capelin, menhaden, anchovetta, or cod)*.
- Goat's milk *(preferably unpasteurized)*.
- Goat cheese *(preferably unpasteurized)*.
- Goat kefir *(preferably unpasteurized)*.
- Goat yogurt.

AFTERNOON SNACK IDEAS

Daily Essentials
- 1/2 liter *(quart)* of water mixed with 1/2 tablespoon of MSM crystals.

Raw Choices
- 2 cucumbers.
- 2 ribs of celery or bok choy.
- One papaya or bowl of fresh figs.
- One appetizer bowl of olives.
- Dehydrated crackers.
- 1 handful of hemp seeds.
- 1 handful of macadamia nuts.
- A young coconut.

(Please reference the raw-food recipe books, Raw Transformation and Rawvolution, for unique snack ideas)

Heated or Cooked Choices
- Popcorn made with cold-pressed coconut oil.
- Baked, no-salt corn chips with guacamole *(avocado, cilantro, olives, lime juice, tomatoes, onions, celtic sea salt, etc.)*

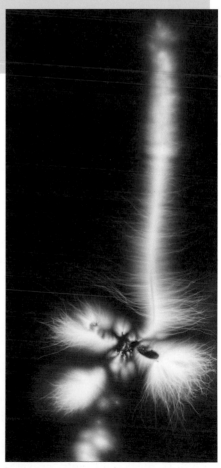

Young Wheatgrass — Blade and Roots
(Kirlian Image)

DINNER IDEAS

Daily Essentials
- 1/2 liter (quart) of fresh vegetable juice containing at least 60% green vegetables, 40% other vegetables or fruits (apple, cucumber, etc.).
- One large leafy-green salad (see Lesson 10: Beauty Recipes under Salads for ideas).

Raw Choices
- Gourmet raw-food (see Lesson 10: Beauty Recipes under Gourmet Menu for ideas).
- Dessert (see Lesson 10: Beauty Recipes under Desserts for ideas).
- Sprouted bread (Essene bread is a dehydrated, no-yeast, flat bread made from sprouted grains).
- One cup of nettle or chaparral tea (after dinner or before sleep as a nightcap).
- Raw soup (see Lesson 10: Beauty Recipes under Soups for ideas).

Heated or Cooked Choices
- Toasted whole-grain bread (kamut bread, spelt bread) with cold-pressed coconut oil.
- Steamed vegetables (cauliflower, broccoli, asparagus, etc.).
- Steamed artichoke hearts (the best of all cooked foods).
- Brown rice (turmeric powder can be used on this meal).
- Baked yam (turmeric powder can be used on this meal).
- Baked sweet potato (turmeric powder can be used on this meal).
- Tofu (Not a beautifying food, but high in protein. Select only soy products that are NOT genetically modified. Genetically modified foods contain irregular DNA and enzyme inhibitors that may have long-term damaging effects on our health.)
- Rice (or bean) burrito containing lettuce, onions, lime juice, and tomatoes.
- Hummus with fresh vegetables and vegetable fruits (celery, broccoli, cauliflower, cucumbers and tomatoes).
- Vegetable soup (containing more mineral-rich vegetables and less carrots and potatoes).

Animal-Based Foods
- Smoked fish (only from clean, organic sources — not herring, capelin, menhaden, anchovetta, or cod).
- Young, organic, free-range, or wild game (turkey, quail, wild birds, venison, etc.).

Supplement Program

The essence of this book and the raw-nutrition message is that we should receive our nutrients naturally from whole raw-plant-foods. Supplements are secondary and supportive assistants.

The following supplements are actually superfoods, and have the ability to increase the vital force of one or more body systems. Like introducing any new food, one should do it gradually and observe how the body responds. One can gradually, then rapidly, increase the quantity of intake according to one's ability to enjoy them.

MSM — MSM is not truly a supplement, but rather a necessary molecular food, like H_2O. Add 1-3 tablespoons of MSM crystals each day into your morning and afternoon water. If the taste of MSM overpowers the water, you put too much in (a teaspoon of MSM per liter of water will usually be below the taste threshold). MSM potentiates (increases the absorption of) all food nutrients and supplements taken within 12 hours after its consumption.

Whole-Food Vitamin C Powder — Add 2-3 tablespoons each day into a smoothie. Whole-food Vitamin C sources include acerola, amla, and/or camu camu berries. Vitamin C is a wonderful tissue rebuilder, blood-purifier, antioxidant, and immune system enhancer. It works in conjunction with MSM.

Blue Mangosteen (Medicinal Antioxidants) — 2-4 capsules per day. "Medicinal antioxidants" means that this remarkable product contains xanthone antioxidants that are known to have powerful anti-viral, anti-microbial, and anti-fungal properties. This is one of the few antioxidant products on the market created with 100% organic ingredients and without chemical solvent extraction. Take 6-8 capsules before heavy sun exposure or airline travel to protect you from UV rays.

Tocotrienols — 1-2 tablespoons a day. This is the most potent form of antioxidant vitamin E available. Great to include in smoothies. This raw extract of rice at one time was priced at $4,000 a tub, now, due to technological advances, it is about $50 a tub.

Silica (*select one or more of the following three silica sources for your personal program*):

Sunfood Nutrition's Ormus Gold (*containing silica*) — 1-2 droppers full per day taken sublingually. This product is a very special mineral supplement that took me over ten years to formulate. This product is made from 99.999% pure gold and silica.

Orgono (*Living Silica*) — This is one of the more powerful healing products on the market. Suffice to say, this silica is miraculous. It comes to you in the form of an ionized liquid silica water.

Vegetal Silica — 1-3 capsules per day. This is a water-soluble, aqueous extract of the herb, spring horsetail. Flora's Silica supplement is formulated using the method designed by Nobel-prize nominee Louis Kervran, author of *Biological Transmutations*. This supplement improves the strength of the bones, hair, skin, and nails.

Sun Is Shining Superfood — 1-3 tablespoons each day. This is one of the best powdered green food blends in the world. *Sun Is Shining Superfood* is so full of natural alkaline minerals and nutrients that it diminishes the appetite and increases energy.

Pure Synergy — 1-3 tablespoons each day. This is the original green superfood blend developed by my friend Mitchell May to help himself recover from a serious car accident in which he nearly lost his leg. Pure Synergy contains superior-quality and high quantity proteins. This organic powder can be added to smoothies, coconut water, purified water, juices, etc.

Chaparral — This herb can be made into a cold tea by placing chaparral leaves in water for 1-4 hours. Start with a very, very mild cold tea. Experiment with this herb and determine what is the best concentration for you. The more you drink chaparral water/tea, the more the taste will grow on you. If boiled into a strong tea, chaparral can be too intense. Chaparral contains molybdenum. This trace mineral enhances hemoglobin formation and helps with the assimilation of MSM. Chaparral is a great balancer to MSM and vitamin C. I recommend a small glass (*8 fluid ounces*) of chaparral tea each day when possible.

Goji Berries — Goji berries are considered the number one food/herb in the entire 5,000 year history and 8,000 herb Chinese medicinal system. Generally considered a tonic longevity food, goji berries deserve at least a mention as a beauty food with their extraordinary content of protein (*18 amino acids*) and beta carotene (*#1 of any food*). Goji berries are often found in Chinese herbal beauty formulas for women along with schizandra berries (*a superherb*), dried longans, pearls (*powdered — a great source of the right kind of calcium*) and angelica root (*dong quai*). Goji berries may be eaten, made into hot tea, simply soaked in water as a cold tea, or powdered and mixed with other herbs as mentioned above.

Beauty Enzymes™ — 1 to 3 capsules with every meal, depending on the size of the

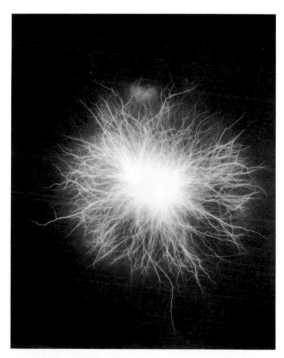

Chaparral Leaf (Kirlian Image)

meal. The more cooked food in the meal, the more enzymes are to be taken. This is the most advanced and comprehensive enzyme formula ever developed. Tested to be 7 times more potent than most enzymes on the market and twice as powerful as the next-best formula. These enzymes are 100% plant-based, natural, non-GMO *(not genetically modified)*, and certified kosher. They improve the digestive breakdown of foods, increase assimilation of nutrients, clean the blood, soften and eradicate internal and external scar tissue, and purify the organs *(including the skin)*. Preferably, they are taken at the start of the meal — though one benefits even if one takes them after eating. They can also be taken between meals to help with weight loss and detoxification. If one has an ulcer, sprinkle them onto the food, let them sit for few minutes, allowing the food to predigest, before beginning the meal. If one is a hemophiliac, on immune suppressant drugs, or has ulcers, then enzymes should not be used between meals. Enzymes help with weight loss by increasing the efficiency of digestion. They may be taken even if one is eating 100% raw-food. They greatly help digest raw, unsprouted nuts and seeds.

Probiotics — Probiotics *(beneficial bacteria)* may be taken with or between meals. Probiotics include bacteria such as: acidophilus, bifidus, bulgaricus, plantarum, salivarius, and many others. It is better to avoid taking them with starchy meals *(bread, pasta, rice, corn chips, etc.)*. Start with 1 capsule with each meal. Probiotics help facilitate weight loss by greatly improving the intestinal environment, allowing for better digestion, assimilation, and elimination.

Weight Loss Program

Remember: The best cleansing and weight loss strategy is to stay positive, do the best you can, work toward eating at least 80% raw-plant-food, and adopt one cleansing program at a time.

The raw-food diet plan provided in this book will be helpful with the weight loss and cleansing process. In addition to these, the following cleansing products are great to add to your weight-loss program, especially when you first begin with raw-food nutrition:

7-Day Raw-Food Weight Loss Plan

This 7-day weight-loss plan works best when used while eating 100% raw-foods for 3 meals each day, 7 days in a row. In addition to raw-plant-food, during the 7-day plan, only enzymes, probiotics, *Sun Is Shining Superfood* or *Pure Synergy*, and water *(with MSM powder)* are included in the diet.

Daily Supplement Intake for the 7-Day Weight-Loss Cleanse

Enzymes — 1 to 3 with meals, 1 to 2 between meals, and 1 to 2 at around 3 am *(if you can get up at that time!)*.

Probiotics — 1 to 2 between meals, and 1 to 3 at bedtime.

MSM — add one teaspoon of MSM crystals *(powder)* to each liter of water you drink.

Sun Is Shining Superfood or Pure Synergy — 3-6 tablespoons with a coconut water or fruit smoothie in the morning. If possible, add 1-2 tablespoons of coconut oil to this smoothie *(to help speed up metabolism)*. The high mineral and protein content of these powdered superfoods helps to cleanse toxins without making you feel depleted or weak and helps to balance the sugar in fruit *(essentially, these superfoods decrease sugar highs and lows)*.

Remember to start with small dosages and increase slowly throughout the week. These supplements may be taken together when appropriate.

Recall that the two major food groups to limit and/or eliminate from the diet in order to lose weight are:

1. Cooked starches. This includes: baked potatoes, rice, beer, bread, pasta, corn chips, potato chips, etc. These foods have

a high glycemic index (they contain a high amount of sugar — starch is turned into sugar when heated). If this sugar is not used by the body, it is converted into fat. Those who excessively eat these types of foods and do not exercise will accumulate layers of fat under the dermal surface in the form of cellulite.

2. Cooked fat. This includes: high-fat meats (bacon, hot dogs, etc.), cooked oil, soy products, pasteurized dairy products, and roasted nuts. Cooked fat is very difficult for the body to metabolize because it is not miscible with water. Stores of undigested cooked fats are retained by the body in the form of flab and plaque deposits in the arteries. Stored fat becomes most noticeable as cellulite on the legs and tummy area.

Remember to drink twice as much water as normally recommended while cleansing. As mentioned previously, take your total weight *(in pounds)* and divide it by four. This will give a number. This number is then the approximate number of fluid ounces of water one should drink in a day. For example, let's say you weigh 120 pounds. 120 divided by 4 is 30. A good daily intake of water is then 30 ounces *(a little less than a 32-ounce quart)*. *(One fluid ounce is equivalent to approximately 30 milliliters)*. While cleansing, it would be wise to increase from 30 ounces to 60 ounces *(double)*.

Other Cleansing and Weight Loss Programs

EJUVA Cleanse — A complete month-long, 100% raw, herbal cleansing program. This is highly recommended once one has been on The Beauty Diet® for six months to a year.

EJUVA Parasite Cleanse — Everyone should do a parasite cleanse at some point. This flush consists of various herbs that are added to the daily routine.

EJUVA Candida Cleanse — This is another pervasive and increasing problem that is related to a systemic weakened body condi-

tion created by a lifetime of consuming too many carbohydrates, antibiotics, and "weak" domesticated foods of all types. This cleanse herbally addresses at least three different types of candida.

Remember: Do one type of cleanse at a time. Take several weeks, or even months, between cleanses to allow your body to come back to homeostasis. Everything should come about in its own time. Too much at once is other than excellent.

Topical Treatments: Food For The Skin

Below, I have listed the most simple effective topical treatments I have discovered. I personally use all of them.

MSM Lotion — The magic of MSM in this Sunfood Nutrition topical skin formula continues to impress individuals year after year. From poison oak/ivy treatment to simple wrinkle-fighting anti-aging skin nutrition, Sunfood Nutrition's MSM Lotion delivers.

Coconut Butter/Oil
(see Lesson 8: Beautifying Foods)

Cacao Butter — Raw chocolate oil is now possible. For the first time ever, Sunfood Nutrition (www.sunfood.com) has made cacao butter *(cocoa butter)* available in its raw form. Cacao butter can be used over every part of your skin. In fact, nothing is better for one's lips and the delicate areas around the eyes where pores are small. Cacao butter smells and tastes like chocolate, because it is chocolate! For liberal use.

Stone-Crushed Olive Oil
(see Lesson 8: Beautifying Foods)

— How To Use These — Topical Treatments

Each evening, after a warm bath or shower *(and after drying)*, massage one of the above mentioned topical treatments into your skin. Let the treatment soak in for twenty minutes and then towel off any remaining oils. You may rotate these treatments around on different days; then leave a day or two — or even longer — with nothing on your skin.

Remember to have your massage therapist use coconut oil on your skin each session.

Keep in mind that your own water-based sprays *(i.e. rose water spray, etc.)* may be used more frequently than other topical treatments. These products are fantastic for those with oily skin.

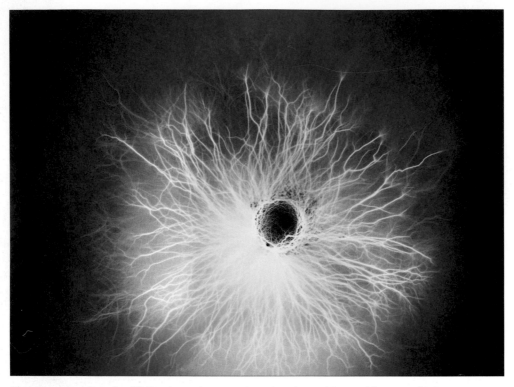

Raw Chocolate Powder *(Kirlian Image)* — raw chocolate (cacao) is good for your skin!

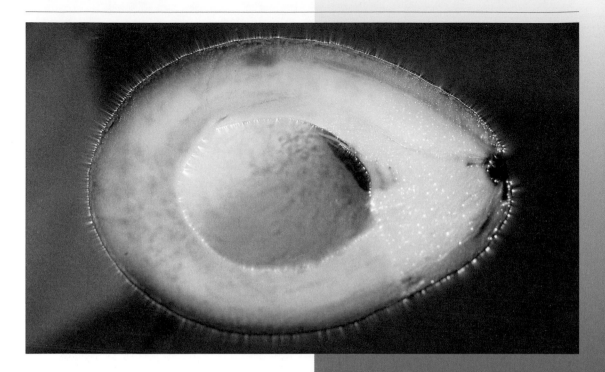

BEAUTY RECIPES

$\mathcal{Ol}$ recommend that you bring several different raw-food recipe books into your kitchen in order to give you unique ideas and variety. I recommend the following books:

Raw Transformation
by Wendy Rudell

RAW
by Roxanne Klein and Charlie Trotter

Rawvolution
by Matt Amsden

Raw: The Uncook Book
by Juliano

The recipes in this section have all been perfected by gourmet raw-food chef, David "Pepperman" Steinberg.

About The Recipes

Avocados are included in many recipes. They are truly a beautifying food in their own right. They are more beautifying when purchased ripe at farmers' markets or picked underneath wild trees, since the oil and minerals will have been allowed to mature properly, because the avocados sat on the trees for an appropriate longer duration.

Cashews are included in the Gourmet Menu section. They are one of the most concentrated sources of zinc found in any food. Like macadamia nuts, they are also rich in beautifying oleic fatty acids. If they are actually raw, I consider them a beautifying food. Because nearly all cashews are steamed and cracked through excessive heat, even if they are labeled raw, they are not. The only truly raw cashews available in North America are distributed by www.sunfood.com.

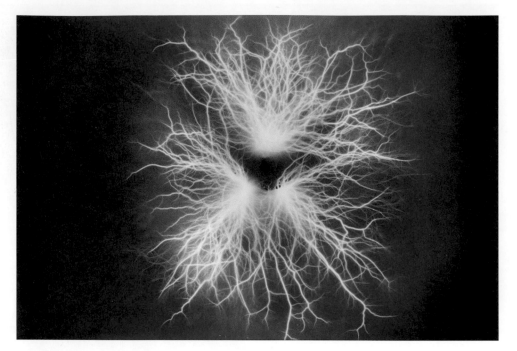

Goji Berry *(Kirlian Image)*

Recall that all ingredients in our diet should be organically grown.

For soups, dressings, and other recipes requiring blending, I recommend the use of a high-powered blender, such as a Vita-mix.

Salads

Hair-Building Salad
(Zinc & Vitamin A Salad)

Arugula . . . . .1 pound (1/2 kg)

Watercress . . . . .1 pound (1/2 kg)

Hair-Building Salad Dressing

Poppy seeds
(soaked for 6 hours, drained) . . . . . .2 tablespoons

Pumpkin seeds
(soaked for 6 hours, drained) . . . . . .2 tablespoons

Water . . . . .1 cup

Parsley (chopped) . . . . .1/2 cup

Celtic Grey Mineral Sea Salt . . . . . . .1/2 tablespoon

Lemon juice .1 lemon

Arrange the greens attractively on a serving platter. Blend all dressing ingredients from low to high, until smooth. An option is to add some of the salad greens

to the dressing. Pour a "living river" of dressing across the center of the salad. If desired, garnish with parsley, celery leaves, sliced black radish, red bell peppers, and sprinkle with unsoaked poppy and pumpkin seeds. Serves: 4.

Skin-Glow Sulfur Salad

Arugula . . . . .1.5 pounds
(3/4 kg)

Watercress . . . . .1 pound (1/2 kg)

Lacinto "dinosaur" kale
(finely diced) . . . . .3 leaves

Celery "hearts" *(sliced)* . . . . .1 cup

Skin-Glow Sulfur Salad Dressing

Tomatoes . . . . .3 medium

Cucumber *(with skin)* . . . . .1 medium

Water . . . . .1/2 cup

Rosemary *(chopped)* . . . . .1 tablespoon

Thyme *(stemmed)* . . . . .1 tablespoon

Sunfood Nutrition Italian olives 6

Sunfood Nutrition Moroccan olives .6

Sunfood Nutrition Moroccan olive water
(from the olive jar) . . . . .2 tablespoons

Garlic . . . . .1 clove

Combine salad ingredients in a large bowl. Blend the dressing without the olives until smooth. Add the olives and blend again until smooth. Add the dressing to the salad, mix thoroughly, and serve. If desired, garnish with zucchini, sliced green onions, and diced red bell pepper. Serves: 3.

Silicon Beauty Salad

Silicon creates beautiful, elastic skin. It remedies brittle fingernails and keeps the hair from turning prematurely gray. Silicon also relieves the pain of tendonitis and related ligament inflammation.

Salad

Romaine lettuce *(chopped)* . . . .1 head
Cucumbers, pickling
   (sliced with skin) 4
Okra *(sliced)* 6
Nopales *(finely diced)* 2
Radishes *(sliced)* 4
Burdock root *(sliced with skin)* . . .1
Tomatoes 4
Red bell peppers *(diced)* 2

Silicon Beauty Salad Dressing

Nettles *(whole leaf, dried)* . . . . . .1 tablespoon
Stone-crushed extra-virgin
   olive oil . . . . .1/3 cup
Lemon juice . . . . .1 lemon
Lime juice . . . . .1 lime
Garlic *(with the skin)* . . . . .1 clove
Italian parsley . . . . .1/4 bunch
Basil . . . . 4 leaves

Combine salad ingredients in a large bowl. Blend the dressing ingredients, low to high, until completely smooth and creamy. Add the dressing to the salad, mix, and serve. Garnish with fennel, dill, rosemary, and lemon twists! Garlic, with the skin, is used in this dressing and several others, because the skin and the area just under the skin contain unique flavors, as well as powerful immune-system boosting elements.
Serves: 4.

Skin-Saver Salad

Radish, red or black
(cut in half-moon slices) 4
Arugula . . . . .1 pound (1/2 kg)
Pinenuts . . . . .1/3 cup
Avocado *(diced)* 1
Garlic *(finely diced)* . . . . .1 clove

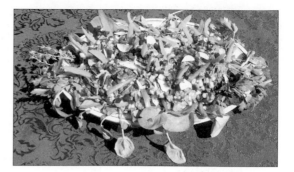

Lemon juice . . . . .1 lemon
Yellow squash or sunburst squash
(finely diced) . . . . .1 medium
Parsley *(finely diced)* . . . . .1/2 bunch
Sunfood Nutrition Italian olives
(chopped) . . . . .1/2 jar

Combine all ingredients. Toss thoroughly. Serve on a beautiful platter. Garnish with herbs, julienned cucumbers, diced red peppers, and julienned yellow peppers. Pine nuts contain a high quantity of MSM.
Serves: 2.

Papaya Fruit Salad

Papaya 1
Avocado 1/2
Fresh figs 6
Nectarines .2
Cinnamon .1/2 tablespoon
Lemon juice . . . . .1 lemon
Raw honey .1 tablespoon

Chop all ingredients, mix, and serve.

Eating this fruit salad is a great way to begin the morning if you do well with carbohydrates and fats. The cinnamon contains the mineral chromium, a great blood-sugar balancer. This fruit salad is loaded with enzymes to help stimulate bowel elimination in the morning.

Dressings
Basic Raw Salad Dressing

Stone-crushed olive oil . . . . .1 cup
Lemon juice or
   Raw apple cider vinegar . . . . . . .1/2 cup
Dried figs, dates, or honey . . . . .1 tablespoon of
                                honey, or 2 dates
                                or dried figs

Blend up a combination of these three types of ingredients. Use this recipe as a basis for building more complex dressings. The olive oil aids digestion. The acids in the lemon juice or vinegar help to break down vegetable fibers. The dried fruit or honey adds sweetness to the mix. You may notice that these three types of ingredients *(an oil, an acid, and a sweetener)* are typically used in cooked, commercial salad dressings.

Italian Dressing

Basic Raw Salad Dressing	*(see previous page)*
Basil, fresh	1 cup
Thyme, fresh *(just leaves, de-stemmed)*	1/2 cup
Rosemary	4 sprigs
Garlic (with skin)	1 clove

Blend the Basic Raw Salad Dressing with the additional ingredients until smooth.
Serves: 2-4.

Indian Curry

Basic Raw Salad Dressing	*(see previous page)*
Turmeric powder	2 tablespoons
Cilantro *(chopped)*	1 tablespoon
Parsley	1/4 bunch
Garlic *(with skin)*	1 clove
Ginger	1 inch (2.5 cm) piece
Celtic Grey Mineral Sea Salt	2 tablespoons
Hot chili pepper *(diced)*	1

Blend the Basic Raw Salad Dressing with the additional ingredients until smooth.
Serves: 2-4.

Mexican Dressing

Basic Raw Salad Dressing	*(see previous page)*
Cilantro	1 cup
Parsley	1/4 bunch
Garlic (with skin)	1 clove
Hot chili pepper	1
Rosemary (diced)	2 tablespoons
Lime juice	1 lime
Cumin seed (freshly ground)	1.5 tablespoons
Tomatoes (ripe)	2 medium
Avocado	1 large

Blend the Basic Raw Salad Dressing with the additional ingredients, except the avocado, until smooth. Add the avocado, blend again.
Serves: 2-4.

Soups
Antioxidant Soup

Arugula	1/2 pound (1/4 kg)
Parsley	1 bunch
Turmeric	1 inch (2.5 cm) slice
Red onion	1/3
Lemons	2
Avocado	1
Sunfood Nutrition Moroccan olives *(pitted)*	6
Tomato	1 medium
Yellow bell peppers	2
Dulse strips	1 handful of
Celtic Grey Mineral Sea Salt	1/2 teaspoon
Unpasteurized miso	1 tablespoon
Hempseed oil	3 tablespoons
Pumpkin seeds	20
Dill	1/4 cup

Shave the outer skin of the lemons, leaving the bioflavonoid-rich white pith and seeds intact. While blending all ingredients, add pure water to reach a thick, soupy consistency.
Serves: 4-6.

Juices & Smoothies
Beauty Beverage

Romaine lettuce	1 head
Cucumber *(with skin)*	1 large
Burdock root *(with skin)*	1
Apple	1

Process all ingredients through your juice machine.
Serves: 2.

Sun Is Shining Superfood Smoothie

Young coconuts *(water and flesh)*	2
Coconut oil *(cold-pressed)*	3 tablespoons
Sun Is Shining Superfood	3 tablespoons
Hemp seeds	3 tablespoons
Dried Calimyrna figs	4

Blend all ingredients to a smooth consistency and serve.
Serves: 3.

Papaya Smoothie

Papaya
(with seeds and skin removed) 1
Sun Is Shining Superfood . . . . .2 tablespoons
Mango 1
Avocado 1/2

Blend all ingredients to a smooth consistency and serve.
Serves: 3.

Airline Rescue Smoothie

Whole-food vitamin C powder . . . .4 tablespoons
Sun Is Shining Superfood . . . . .3 tablespoons
Orange juice . . . . .2/3 liter (quart)
Hempseed oil . . . . .3 tablespoons
Stabilized oxygen supplement
(in liquid) . . . . .3 droppers full
Spring Water . . . . .1 cup

Blend all ingredients to a smooth consistency and serve.
The oxygen supplement is available in your healthfood
store under various brands. This drink helps you rejuvenate from long airflights.
Serves: 2.

Grapefruit Cellulite Reduction Cocktail

Grapefruit *(pink)* . . . . .3 large
Orange . . . . .1 large
Lemon
(Ponderosa is the best variety) 1
                                        medium
Feijoa *(pineapple guava)* 4

Slice all fruits in half and process through a citrus juicer. Feijoas are scarce in most areas of
North America. If you cannot find them, add 1
cup of fresh pineapple juice instead. This is a
great drink for cellulite reduction! Fast on this
drink for three days and see miracles happen.
Serves: 4.

Desserts
Erotic Cream

This recipe goes well with sliced whole fruit.

Honey dates
*(pitted, soaked in orange juice
overnight, drained)* 8
Calimyrna figs
*(soaked in orange juice
overnight, drained)* 8

Dried cranberries
*(soaked in 3 oz. apple juice
overnight, drained)* . . . . .3 ounces
                                        (90 grams)
Currants *(soaked in orange juice
overnight, drained)* . . . . .2 ounces
                                        (60 grams)
Fresh orange juice
*(you may use the O.J. drained
from the dates)* . . . . .4 ounces
                                        (120 grams)
Macadamia nuts *(raw, shelled)* . . . .1 cup
Cacao nibs
(raw chocolate pieces) . . . . .1/2 cup
Vanilla bean *(slice lengthwise
and scrape out inside)* 1
Young coconut
(water and soft flesh) 1
Celtic Grey Mineral Sea Salt . . . . . . .1 pinch

Blend (from low to high): coconut water, dates, cranberries, and currants until smooth. Add macadamia
nuts and coconut flesh, blend from low to high until
smooth. Serve. Perfect erotic nutrition for you and your
partner.
Serves: 2.

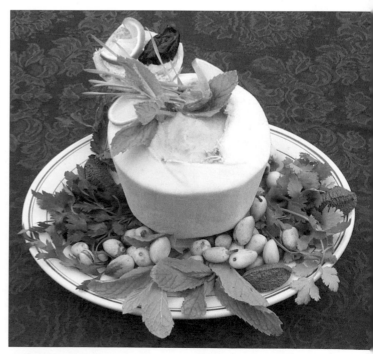

Erotic Cream

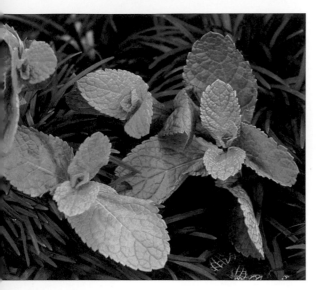

Fresh Mint

Raw Ice Cream

Frozen bananas 6

Frozen blueberries . . . . .1 cup

Papaya 1

Mint leaves .3-4

Blueberries contain a high concentration of antioxidants in their blue color. Run the bananas and blueberries through a Champion or Green Life juicer with the solid plate in place. This will create a soft-serve ice cream. Add papaya pieces and garnish with mint.
Serves: 4.

Gourmet Menu

Raw gourmet chef, David "Pepperman" Steinberg, has unleashed five of his most incredible gourmet raw-food recipes for this section.

These awesome recipes quite simply reach a new plateau of taste explosion, while remaining easy to assemble and, of course, are 100% raw and organic. All diced vegetable quantities are measured AFTER dicing. If maple syrup is not obtained fresh as maple water, it is cooked. You may choose another sweetener, such as honey or blended dates and water as a substitute.

The Pepperman's Bread-n-Buddha Cheese

This creamy, yet crunchy cheese actually tastes exactly like fresh French bread and garlic slathered with creamy butter. Wow!

Cheese

Sunfood Nutrition cashews
(soaked & drained overnight) . . .1 pound (1/2 kg)

Lemon juice . . . . .2 lemons

Lemon zest (diced yellow
outer lemon peel) . . . . .1 lemon

Lime juice .1 lime

Celtic Grey Mineral Sea Salt . . . .2 teaspoons

Garlic (pressed or finely diced) . .2 cloves

Dulse (flakes or powder) . . . . .1 tablespoon

Run cashews through a Champion Juicer or Green Life juicer with the blank attachment assembled. Add remaining ingredients. Stir thoroughly with wooden spoon. Beat with wooden spoon for 2 minutes to infuse garlic and oxygenate the cheese! Transfer to a smaller wooden or glass bowl and place uncovered in the dehydrator at 100 degrees Fahrenheit for 24-36 hours. Longer dehydration times result in more pronounced flavor, as well as a more crusty texture. Stirring every 4 hours is recommended. Enjoy! (This recipe will last over 10 days in the refrigerator).
Serves: 6.

The Pepperman's Cosmic Cashew Yogurt

This "I can't believe it's not dairy" yogurt is a thick, rich, creamy gift from raw-food heaven. You'll swear it's real yogurt (except you will know it is better!).

To make flavored yogurts, simply add fresh berries, peaches, or any fresh fruit desired. Always drink one coconut out of each box before using the others in recipes to gauge the sweetness of the batch.

Yogurt

Coconut water . . . . .2 young Thai

Coconut "meat" . . . . .4 young Thai

Hemp seeds . . . . .1/3 cup

Sunfood Nutrition cashews
(soaked overnight & drained) . . .1/3 cup

Pure, unfiltered organic
maple syrup . . . . .3 tablespoons

Fresh vanilla bean
(soft inside seeds) . . . . .1 whole

Coconut oil (cold-pressed) . . . . .2 tablespoons

Lemon juice . . . . .2 lemons

Combine fresh sweet coconut water from one coconut with all of the coconut "meat." Blend. Be sure to

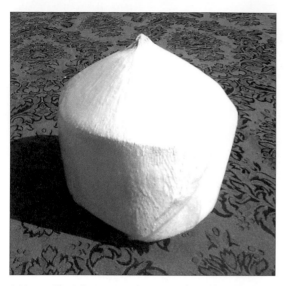

A Young Thai Coconut as it appears in Asian Markets
(This type of coconut has had the outer green husk shaved off).

include absolutely NO bits of coconut shell whatsoever. This will alter the beautiful white color and creamy texture of the finished product. Blend this mixture on low, then gradually raise to high, until thoroughly blended. Avoid over-mixing, scrape sides with spatula. Add remaining ingredients. Blend again low to high. Use some of the remaining coconut water to thin out yogurt, if needed. Store in fridge.
Serves: 4.

To make mayonnaise: Replace coconut water with pure water. Add 1 tablespoon of celtic salt, 1 small clove of garlic, and 1/2 teaspoon cayenne.

Red-Hot-Pepper-Powerman's Tasmanian Tandori Cucumber Salad & Oil-Free Dressing

Conjuring up flavors and textures of Chinese, Mexican, and Thai cuisine, this dish is really an Indian-inspired

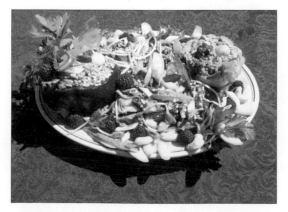

masterpiece delivering incomprehensible beneficial properties too numerous to list here.

Salad

Pickling cucumbers *(cut on bias)*	3 medium
Yellow squash *(cut on bias)*	3 small
Red onion *(thin half moons)*	1 medium
Young coconut "meat" *(harder the better), (diced)*	2 "meats"
Romaine *(core & end part)*	1 cup
Broccoli *(finely diced & including stems)*	1 cup
Arugula *(chopped)*	1 cup
Celery "heart" *(diced)*	1 bunch
Bread-n-Buddha cheese	1 cup
Sunflower greens	2 cups
Cashews	1 cup

To cut on a "bias," simply cut cucumbers in half lengthwise, place cut side down, cut 2 times lengthwise (horizontally), then chop from top to bottom diagonally. Presto — nifty, raw cucumber diamonds! Chop crisp Romaine very small. Mix all ingredients in large wood or glass bowl. Place 1/2 cup of the Bread-n-Buddha Cheese in each of two sliced and hollowed bell peppers. Garnish with sunflower greens and cashews.

Oil-Free Dressing

Spring water	1-2 cups
Cucumbers *(chopped)*	1 whole
Italian parsley	large handful
Curly parsley	small handful
Dill	small handful
Fennel *(diced)*	1/3 cup
Basil	tender leaves only
Rosemary (chopped)	2 tablespoons
Lemon juice	3 lemons
Lime juice	1 lime
Celtic Grey Mineral Sea Salt	1 tablespoon
Italian olives *(diced)*	8 each
Moroccan olives *(pitted, chopped)*	8 each
Okra	3 pod-fruits, diced
Garlic *(with skin)*	2 large cloves
Ginger *(diced small)*	1 inch (2.5 cm) piece
Red hot pepper *(diced)*	1 whole
Large avocado *(ripe, still firm)*	1 whole
Cumin powder *(organic)*	3 tablespoons

Turmeric powder (organic) . . . . .1 tablespoon

Watercress . . . . .small handful

Black radish (diced) (use red
or daikon if black is out) . . . . .1/3 cup

Maple syrup or raw honey . . . . . .1/3 cup

Blend all except olives and avocado. When completely blended, add olives. Blend to incorporate, then add avocado. Should be ultra green-creamy, like soup. Mix 1-2 cups with salad. Serve. Leave the remaining dressing on the side. Serves: 4.

Pepperman's High-Powered Papaya Pudding

This incredibly quick, super-easy recipe uses the pre-made Cosmic-Cashew Yogurt to yield an unbelievably silky-smooth pudding, which can be used as a pie filling. This is an integral component of layered custard desserts, frozen "sorbets," or smoothies.

Pudding

Large papaya . . . . .4 to 6 lbs. (3 cups
after scooping)

Dried apricots (soaked
overnight & drained) . . . . .1/3 cup

Cosmic Cashew Yogurt . . . . .1 cup

Chocolate mint leaves (diced) . .2 tablespoons

Coconut oil (cold-pressed) . . . . .2 tablespoons

The idea here is to blend all ingredients thoroughly and completely, while preserving the delicate texture of the papaya. Using the yogurt puts us a step ahead, by having the ingredients within it already blended. Be attentive — use the blender's speed control knob and blend just enough to achieve smoothness, and that's it! Combine all ingredients except coconut oil, scrape sides with spatula and make sure the mint is blended. Next blend in coconut oil on low-medium speed. Serve in papaya shell. Decorate with berries, orange slices, chocolate mint, and spearmint. Impeccable! Serves: 4.

Interplanetary Okra Salad & Astral Beauty Dressing

This stunning green salad earned its name by causing first-time eaters to be transported to "other worlds," where limitations on shockingly high taste and enzyme extremes simply don't exist. Flavors intensify over time, yet salad may become soggy if saved for longer than one day. It has never lasted longer than one hour at our raw-food headquarters!

Salad

Okra (sliced thin on bias) . . . . . . .7 pod-fruits

Romaine (core end pieces) . . . . .1-2 cups

Arugula (chopped) . . . . .1/2 cup

Celery hearts
(bias cut, Chinese style) . . . . .1 cup

Jerusalem artichoke
(finely diced) . . . . .1/2 cup

Cucumber (pickling) . . . . .1 medium

Red bell pepper
(finely diced) . . . . .1 whole

Yellow bell pepper (julienned) . . .1 whole

Ripe Tomato, romas
(seeded, julienned) . . . . .4 small

Broccoli (finely diced) . . . . .1 cup

Combine all and toss. Okra is a beautifying food in its own right!

Astral Beauty Dressing

Stone-crushed olive oil . . . . .1 cup

Flaxseed oil . . . . .1/2 cup

Spring water . . . . .1/2 cup

Lemon juice . . . . .1/2 cup

Celtic Grey Mineral Sea Salt . . . .1 tablespoon

Ginger (finely diced) . . . . .1 teaspoon

Garlic (with skin) . . . . .2 medium cloves

Okra (chopped) . . . . .2 pod-fruits

Hemp seeds . . . . .1/3 cup

Red hot chili pepper (diced) . . . .1 whole

Coconut meat (soft) . . . . .1 whole

Blend all except coconut meat. Scrape sides. Add coconut meat and blend till smooth. It should be creamy, yet slightly thin. Toss with salad. Garnish with long, thin okra slices, Italian parsley, celery leaf, and julienned tomato slices! Serves: 4.

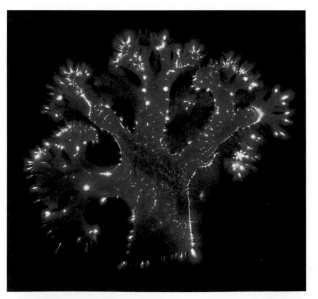

Raw Organic Broccoli (Kirlian Image)

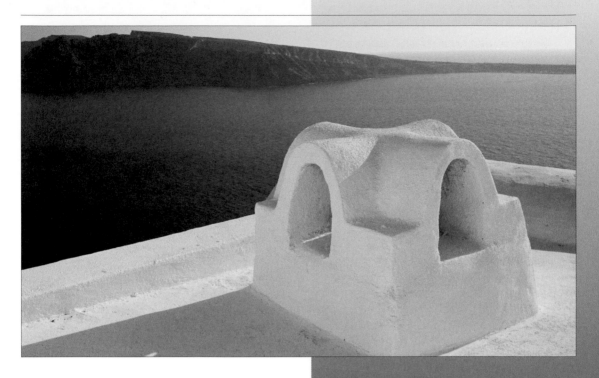

Skin

The color, softness, and texture of the skin are the most important elements of beauty. The skin should radiate exquisite freshness, thus expressing the inner truth of excellent health. Nothing is as attractive as clear, fresh skin.

In order to have soft cheeks and silky, radiant skin, we must choose a lifestyle that is favorable to skin-beauty and natural skin-tinting.

Care of the skin begins with internal cleanliness and proper raw-food choices. Recall that the beauty foods bring vital silicon, sulfur, vitamin A, vitamin C, vitamin E, and an array of antioxidants to the skin. MSM (*methyl-sulfonyl-methane*) also assists in completely rebuilding the skin from the inside. MSM works on multiple levels to rejuvenate the liver and increase nutrient absorption while delivering sulfur to the skin.

The skin is the last organ to be nourished because it is the furthest away from the digestive organs. Because we absorb nutrients

"Skin, Hair, Nails, Teeth, Eyes, Voice"

through our skin, it is important to nourish the skin from both the inside and the outside.

— How The Skin Is Damaged —

Our skin is made supple and beautiful by collagen. Collagen is a long-living protein that is subject to free radical (unstable oxygen) attack. A chemical change in the collagen (*called cross-linking*) due to free radical exposure, leads to hidden inflammation and eventually wrinkles and damaged skin.

Free radical damage causes a change in the lipid characteristics of the outer layer of the epidermis. These lipid characteristics are often improved and healed by applying healing oils such as hemp oil, stone-crushed olive oil, and/or coconut oil directly to the skin daily, if appropriate and necessary. Another option is to do nothing to the skin for several weeks or months in order to let the skin breathe and allow the natural balance to be restored.

The primary causes of free radical collagen damage and skin aging are poor nutrition, internal toxicity, dehydration, overexposure to sunshine, using commercial chemical soaps, smoking, bathing in hard tap water, exposure to extremely dry, cold weather, and fungal invasion.

Facial wrinkles are deepened by the free radicals caused by smoking. Crow's feet wrinkle patterns around the eyes and on the upper lip are indicative of smoking marijuana and/or cigarettes.

Our skins' health depends greatly on the presence and retention of moisture. The epidermis (the top, thin layer of our skin) has the ability to hold on to moisture if we stay properly hydrated by drinking high-quality water and ingesting the proper nutrients.

If the body is toxic, the liver, the blood's filtering system, will be toxic. Instead of filtering and neutralizing the poisons and toxins in the blood, the toxins remain, get circulated through the body, and are deposited primarily into the fatty tissue. The toxic load eventually causes the cells to degenerate and begin to die for lack of oxygen, water, and nutrients. The aging process is thus accelerated. The longer this process continues, the more malnourished the cells become. The long-term effects can again be seen in wrinkled, spotted, leathery, gray, lifeless skin.

Eczema is often the result of the organs being so filled with toxic materials that the body is forced to push excess toxins into the bloodstream, making it necessary to eliminate them through the skin.

Men have thicker skin than women due to the influence of the dominant male hormone testosterone. Also, men produce more oil on their skin than women. These factors make women more like to experience dry and damaged skin.

— Acne —

Acne is mainly caused by a poor fat/oil digestion and assimilation metabolism. This means the liver is not capable of fully metabolizing all the fat and oil entering the system. The skin and the liver reflect each other like a mirror.

A breakout of the skin, acne, is an indicator of problems with the liver — in particular with the processing of fats — especially cooked fats.

Facial and skin acne are almost always associated with eating cooked oil (margarine, hydrogenated oil, cooked polyunsaturated oils, etc.). Cooked oils and margarine are probably the most difficult of all cooked foods to break down and metabolize. They require a significant level of liver energy. Cooked oils and margarine are often incompletely broken down and end up clumping up in the blood stream, clogging fine capillaries, causing hormonal imbalances, and acne.

Along with cooked oil and margarine, the intake of cooked animal fats, roasted nuts and seeds, as well as pasteurized dairy products can all be decreased, and then eliminated. Raw-plant-based fats and oils can replace cooked fats and oils. This will do wonders.

Even when one is eating raw-foods, one may find that the excessive intake of raw fats and oils will cause pimples (yet these will be comparatively minor).

Simultaneously, while the cooked fats and oils are switched to raw choices, the liver may be strengthened by eating green-leafy vegetables, undertaking herbal cleansing and fasting, and adding MSM to the diet.

One thing I have noticed amongst people with chronic acne, breakouts, and trouble with their facial skin, is that they have an unconscious habit of constantly touching and picking at their face. This introduces foreign dirt and oils, thus making the situation worse.

One of the primary ways to maintain healthy facial skin is to avoid touching one's face with the dirty, oily palm surface of the fingers and hands.

If you have troubles with your complexion, pay close attention to any subconscious habits of touching the face. I only touch my face with the back of my hands. As a youth I picked up the habit of immediately using the backside of my hand to itch my face or wipe things from my lips or cheeks. As a result, I have never had acne.

Another major causative factor in acne is thinking too much about a particular relationship. Releasing confined emotions surrounding a past or present relationship can do wonders to rid an individual of acne.

Acne may also be caused by skin damage *(the outer layer of skin may be thickened, which contracts the pores and does not allow them to breathe)*. If this is the case, enzymatic exfoliation *(a papaya mask)* or similar exfoliation treatment will be helpful. Someone with this type of damaged skin should avoid facial exposure to the sun and should also avoid putting oils on the face, as absorption is poor.

On hot days, since the earliest times I can remember, I often ate grapefruits. As a child I began to intuitively rub the inner surface of these fresh grapefruit peels on my face. I have noticed over the years that this not only has a cooling effect, but also a skin cleansing effect. Grapefruit peels make for a great skin cleanser; they lift dirt right off of your skin. The exfoliating, cleansing properties of grapefruit are likely due to alpha-hydroxy acids. Alpha-hydroxy acids are also found in sugar cane and many other fruits.

Emotional issues are often involved with acne. Suppressed anger accentuates an acne condition.

— Soap —

Skin damage can be caused by years of abusing alkaline soaps and other skin products. The excessive use of commercial soaps and shampoos strips away the skin's oil, damages skin pigments, and removes skin moisture, leaving the skin dry, faded, and coarse.

The skin generally thrives at a slight acidic pH. The extreme alkalinity of soaps disrupts this delicate pH balance.

Soap is particularly harsh on people who have dry skin. If you have dry skin, be sure that you avoid washing your face with soap.

According to my research, the idea of soap was developed by the Germans. Long before German civilization developed soap, the Romans, Greeks, Hebrews, Persians, Incas, Mayans, Chinese, Egyptians, Sumerians, Atlanteans, and every other civilization maintained bodily cleanliness without the use of soap.

The advent of soap followed on the heels of a major increase in cooked animal food and cooked oil in the diet. The residues of cooked fat come through the pores as a smelly, thick waxy fluid that is difficult to wash off without soap. Once one switches to a plant-based diet, the oils coming through the skin are purer, have less odor, and are easier to wash off.

The skin is not only a major organ of elimination, but also of assimilation. We should be careful not to put anything onto our skin that we would not eat.

Instead of soap, one can use a Chocolate Skin Rejuvenation Bar. The unique synergy of the finest skin healing and rejuvenation botanicals in this neat product provides an unprecedented skin revitalizing experience. Apply instead of soap and experience a new type of bathing sensation. Use the Chocolate Skin Rejuvenation Bar to achieve even more glow and vibrancy; the bar is great on all of the skin, face, and hair. This is likely the highest-quality, all-natural skin beauty bar ever created. The Chocolate Skin Rejuvenation Bar contains: certified-organic non-GMO soy oil, certified-organic coconut oil, extra-virgin olive oil *(soy, coconut, and olive oils are saponified with retained glycerin)*, 100% pure cacao *(cocoa)* oil/butter, wild-crafted Coral Sea Island tamanu oil, mangosteen powder *(Garcinia mangostana)* and Moroccan Rhassoul Clay. All the ingredients are: cold-processed, 100% natural, GMO free, vegan, bio-degradable, and cruelty free. The Chocolate Skin Rejuvenation Bar may be found by searching at www.sunfood.com.

Diluted lemon juice or diluted raw apple cider vinegar are other simpler soap substitutes. To make a cleansing liquid, add one tablespoon of lemon juice or raw apple cider vinegar to 6-8 fluid ounces *(180-240 ml)* of warm water.

The best book on how to create your own body-care products at home is *Recipes For Beauty* by Katie Spiers.

I do not rely on soaps or soap substitutes. I mainly clean my skin by dry-skin brushing using a moderately-firm, natural-fiber brush, and then rinsing using warm, not hot, purified water or hot springs water. Dry brushing exfoliates dead skin cells and stimulates the lymphatic system.

— Applying Lotions and Oils —
The caution put forth against putting oils directly onto the face is only valid when the skin is very oily, damaged, and/or absorption is poor. As long as the oils are cold-pressed *(raw)* and they agree with the individual, then putting cacao butter *(best choice)*, hemp oil, olive oil, grapeseed oil, or coconut oil onto the face can provide wonderful benefits to the skin without clogging the pores.

— Coconut Oil —
After puberty, the skin produces its own oil that is secreted from millions of sebaceous glands in the skin tissue. This oil contains medium chain fatty acids *(MCFAs) (see Lesson 8: Beautifying Foods: Coconut Oil)*. This oil *(called sebum)* can destroy certain bacteria, fungi, and viruses. Before puberty, one is more susceptible to certain skin conditions such as viral warts.

Unfortunately, most people strip this oil away with harsh soaps and shampoos. This disrupts the skin's natural protective layer and slightly acidic state.

Sunfood Nutrition's Coconut Oil is a phenomenal skin lotion. Because coconut oil contains large quantities of MCFAs, it not only moisturizes and protects the skin, but it also attacks lipid-coated viruses and bacteria on the skin surface. The medium-chain length of the oil allows it to be more easily absorbed than many other oils.

— Grape Seed Oil —
Though given little attention in this book, grapeseed oil is another excellent skin lotion. Grape seed oil, a powerful antioxidant that has excellent bioavailability, helps to cross-link collagen fibers, preventing collagen destruction. Grapeseed oil should be cold-pressed, not solvent extracted.

— Sunshine —
Sunshine on the skin is an essential component of beauty and health. Denser bones, stronger muscles, richer blood, healthier nerves, and greater endurance are created by regular exposure to sunshine.

Let's consider this information, and yet also understand that oversunning, like overeating, is harmful. Oversunning causes free-radical collagen damage to the skin.

Basically, the prevention of sun-skin damage or a sunburn is easy and requires only a little forethought.

First, consider the fairness of your skin. Melanin is the pigment that gives skin its color. More melanin creates darker skin. With more melanin, one is more resistant to the sun-damage caused by ultra-violet radiation.

Second, employ a simple strategy: enjoy only ten minutes exposure to the sun on the first day — five minutes on the front, and five minutes on the back. This should be steadily increased to 30 minutes exposure on the front and 30 minutes on the back. This full hour of sun is sufficient for anyone.

One can use coconut oil on the skin directly before and after sunning. This stops the skin from drying out, and provides some protection.

— Antioxidant Protection —

Even though rich quantities of antioxidants are found in raw-plant-foods, an additional antioxidant supplement is usually recommended.

Antioxidants protect white blood cells from oxidation and help repair sun damage. Antioxidants offer such amazing natural sun protection that you can tell how effective supplemental antioxidants are by how well your skin is protected during sun exposure.

— Dry Skin —

The stratum corneum, the outermost layer of the epidermis, determines to a large degree how much moisture can be retained. This very thin outer layer is composed of dying and dead skin cells held together by fatty substances built out of dietary fats. If the stratum corneum is weakened, this leads to dry skin. The stratum corneum is totally replaced every 30 days; however, as one ages, this process can take up to 50 days.

A deficiency of omega 6 fatty acids has been correlated with atopic eczema, dry skin, scaling and cracking skin, and some forms of acne. Atopic eczema is characterized by low activity in the sweat glands, causing the skin to itch and feel dry. Clinical trials using gamma-linolenic fatty acids *(a powerful type of anti-inflammatory omega 6)* have yielded gradual improvements in atopic eczema and marked improvements in moisturizing dry, cracking, and/or scaling skin. Hemp seeds, hempseed oil, borage seed oil, and primrose oil are fantastic sources of gamma-linolenic fatty acids.

Unique Facts About Sunshine Exposure:

- Vitamin D, which assists in mineralizing the bones, is formed when the skin is exposed to sunshine.
- Sunshine increases the amount of iron in the blood. This creates a more "magnetic" presence, as is evident in the "well-tanned" look.
- USA cancer rates are highest in the northern states with the least sunshine.
- Rates of breast, prostate, ovarian, and colon cancer are lower in people with more sunshine exposure.
- Sunshine exposure may reduce breast cancer up to 30-40%, and ovarian cancer by 80%.
- There are 2,200 sunlight-associated cancer deaths yearly versus 138,000 for the above-mentioned cancers in the USA.
- Sunshine-associated cancers (non-melanoma) increase most where sunscreens are most heavily promoted.
- Sunshine raises positive moods in persons with SAD (seasonal affective disorder).
- Psoriatic skin lesions are reduced by sunshine.
- Direct sun exposure kills most forms of mold, fungus and yeast (athlete's foot, candida, etc.)
- Daily sunshine exposure normalizes hormone levels in women and men.

— Skin Treatments —

Avocado Mask:

For Dry Skin

Puree one ripe avocado with 6-7 drops of a fresh-squeezed ripe orange. Add one tablespoon of hemp oil. Massage this mixture into the face and neck. This mask has excellent effects on any part of the skin. After application, lie down and relax. Rinse off with lukewarm water after 20-30 minutes.

Cucumber Mask:

For Oily Skin

Peel a cucumber. Finely grate it. Lie down, relax, and apply the cucumber to the face and neck. After applying, place a warm towel over the face. Relax for 20-30 minutes. Rinse off.

Aloe Vera Mask,

"The Instant Face Lift": For Tired and/or Sagging Skin

Fillet a small piece of aloe vera, exposing the inner gel. Rub a thick layer of this inner gel over the face and neck. Lie down and relax. This mask may be applied before sleep and left on throughout the night. Rinse with lukewarm water in the morning.

— Burns —

Raw honey both protects and nourishes damaged skin. There have been more than 35 reports in medical journals of raw honey's clinical application in a total of over 600 patients. A study in 1991 compared conventional silver sulfadiazine burn therapy with the topical application of raw honey. In seven days, 91% of the infected burns treated with raw honey were free of infection, while in the sulfadiazine group less than 7% were free of infection. Within 15 days, 87% of the raw honey group was completely healed, whereas only 10% of the sulfadiazine group had healed in that time.

— Razor Bumps —

According to Dr. Nicholas Perricone, M.D., author of *The Wrinkle Cure*, the topical application of alpha hydroxy acids is the most effective treatment for razor bumps, a condition that afflicts over 50% of African-American males who shave. Alpha hydroxy acids are gentle acids that help the skin slough off dead surface cells and diminish inflammation.

— Cracks on the Heels of the Feet —

MSM lotion works wonders in healing annoying cracks on the heels of the feet. It should be applied three or four times daily to the affected area, until the condition subsides.

Hair

Our hair is an agricultural crop that has its roots in the blood-enriched lymphatic soil beneath the skin. The most important aspect of rehabilitating hair is to cleanse, purify, and nourish the body, blood, and lymphatic system. To maintain healthy hair, adequate nutrition and blood flow to the hair roots is necessary. The primary cause of hair loss and premature graying is a lack of nourishment for renewing the living hair follicle.

A deficiency of one trace mineral, tin, can contribute to male pattern baldness. For male pattern baldness, one food stands out strongly due to its extraordinary level of tin: the schizandra berry, the five flavor fruit from Chinese medicine. This tiny fruit is extremely potent, just 30-40 of these berries a day is sufficient.

Just like our bones, organs and muscles, our hair follicles must also receive adequate nutrition. Malnourishment of the hair follicle is primarily caused by the clogging of the fine capillaries with mucus from mucus-forming foods (*pasteurized dairy products, cooked grains [especially wheat], cooked animal fat, and cooked polyunsaturated oils*). If we want a good hairline, the important thing for us to have is excellent circulation to allow nutrients to flow to the hair follicle.

Eating a raw-food-based diet may not be enough to restore damaged hair follicles — our diets must be well-considered, raw, mineral-rich, and nutrient-dense to achieve the extraordinary result we are seeking

Healthy hair requires specific protein-building amino acids and sulfur in the diet because hair is almost entirely made up of protein (*97%*). These can be found in hemp seeds, spirulina, superfood blends such as

Sun Is Shining Superfood and *Pure Synergy*, and eating a wide variety of organic vegetables and their juices. Animal protein is abrasive, inflammatory, and clogging; therefore it is a poor choice as a hair nutrient.

MSM forms the sulfur bonds between proteins. It also increases the assimilation of protein. One of the first things you will discover after taking MSM is that your hair growth will be stronger and more vigorous.

— Gray Hair —

Premature gray hair is caused by a lack of B vitamins, a deficiency of raw fatty acids and trace minerals *(silicon, sulfur, and copper)*. Dr. Ann Wigmore restored her hair from gray back to its original dark color primarily by drinking rejuvelac *(the enzyme-rich, B-vitamin-rich water left over from the process of sprouting grains)*. Rejuvelac can be made at home *(see Dr. Wigmore's books for instructions)*, but is not generally available at stores. Raw sauerkraut and kim-chi are available at stores and they possess many of the same properties as rejuvelac. I recommend the Rejuvenative Foods brand found in the refrigerated section of your natural food store.

— Hair Care —

Morrocco hair-care products present state-of-the-art, organic, 100% uncooked shampoos, conditioners, and a hair spray. These products are made of minerals and herbs and are great for chemically-sensitive individuals. They are non-toxic and non-allergenic and contain no sodium lauryl sulfates. They nourish the skin and follicles from the outside, complementing excellent internal nutrition.

— Facial Hair —

For men, facial hair is of importance too. When I became a raw-foodist, the hair on my face turned to its natural brown/red color whereas before, it had always been dark brown. Since I started including MSM in my morning water, my facial hair now grows with surprising vigor and strength.

There is even an organic shampoo for mustaches and beards *(www.beardshampoo.com)*.

Nails

I gave a health seminar once, and a woman sitting in the front row kept looking at my hands. At the end of the seminar she approached and told me that her mom had always told her that the health of someone's nails was the key indicator of internal health. Luckily my nails were well groomed for that seminar. I have always remembered to clean my nails before every lecture since that day!

The nails truly are an indication of how well we absorb minerals. If nail ailments have set in, such as ingrown, splitting, soft, spotting, or ridged nails, then the mineral-rich The Beauty Diet® will work wonders. Nail health is the result of the proper mixture of the beautifying foods, silica *(Orgono living silica, horsetail extract)*, and MSM.

Fungus under the finger or toenails is an external sign of an internal imbalance of good and bad bacteria in the intestines. It is often an outward manifestation that bad bacteria and fungus rule the internal environment of the body *(or at least did when the infection occurred)*. Someone who has chronic fungal infection under the nails may also have a candida *(yeast overgrowth)* internally. One-half a dropper full of Pau D'Arco alcohol tincture can be droppered on the nail, under the nail *(as best as possible)*, and on the first and second knuckle of the affected finger after the area has been cleaned. The area must then be "painted" with a few drops of DMSO *(dimethyl-sulfoxide)*. DMSO drives the Pau D'Arco deep into the nail and skin *(avoid liberal usage as DMSO can burn when used excessively)*. It will take 3-6 weeks to begin to see noticeable results. As you stay with this topical program you will be able to fight back the fungus and eventually be victorious. Both Pau D'Arco alcohol tincture and DMSO are available in health-food stores.

If you believe you have candida, please track down *(via my website www.thebestdayever.com)* and read *The Spiritual Immune Tonic System*. Some anti-candida advice you can act on immediately is to include *Sun Is Shining Superfood* each and every day *(in quantities* beginning at 1 tablespoon per day and increasing up to 3 tablespoons per day after two months). Also, probiotic capsules should be taken each day, starting with 1 and building up to 6 each day. Add 3,000-5,000 mg of camu camu berry powder to the diet. All high carbohydrate, sugar-based foods, especially dried fruit, seedless fruit, soda, candy, bread, pasta, baked potatoes, potato chips, corn chips, and rice should be eliminated from the diet. Eat nothing sweeter than a hard pear or tart apple. Coconut oil and good-quality avocados should be eaten as primary fat sources. Mercury-free fish and hemp seed should be eaten for protein.

The habit of nail biting is related to an alkaline mineral deficiency and parasites (worms) in the system. In this case I recommend more herbs, green-leafy salads, and a parasite cleanse (again reference via www.thebestdayever.com, The Spiritual Immune Tonic System).

Teeth

> "Investigations have fully established the following facts:
>
> 1. The teeth of wild animals are superior to those of domestic animals.
>
> 2. Animal teeth, on the whole, are superior to human teeth.
>
> 3. The teeth of ancient man were better than those of modern man.
>
> 4. The teeth of contemporary savages are better than those of highly civilized and 'progressive' peoples.
>
> 5. Civilized peoples still living under what we call backward conditions (so-called 'backwards peoples') have better teeth than people in highly civilized regions where they have all the 'blessings' of dentistry and medical 'science.'"
>
> — Dr. Herbert Shelton

It is clear from Dr. Shelton's insight and a perspective of common sense that the most prominent element of tooth decay is the civ-

ilized diet. In particular, the deficiency of alkaline elements (magnesium, iron, and silicon found in rich green foods) in the civilized diet plays a major role, as does the intake of refined carbohydrates and sugars, and even overly eating natural fruit sugars.

Eating highly-mineralized foods, especially vegetables and superfoods (and halting the intake of heavy acid-forming foods and sugars) can halt tooth decay, and in some cases reverse damage (especially in children and teens). Of all natural foods, chewing on wild grasses has the most remarkable teeth-strengthening qualities. I like to eat fibrous vegetables and herbs, such as celery and licorice root, after eating sweet fruit. Fibrous vegetables and herbs clean and naturally brush the teeth.

In particular, silicon-rich supplements and herbs rich in silicon nourish the teeth directly. Including Orgono living silica and horsetail extract as supplements will be beneficial. Adding an herbal tea to your diet that contains: horsetail, nettles, oat straw, alfalfa, and hemp leaf (where legal) will yield excellent results in strengthening bones and teeth.

Our teeth are living, breathing bones. They are permeable — not solid. Even the strong enamel has tiny tubes running through it. These tubes contain a fluid fed by the bloodstream, which nourishes the teeth.

MSM should be included in a teeth-building program as it helps drive more nutrients into the teeth. Sulfur helps build strong enamel.

A contributing factor to poor dietary choices is the presence of bacteria that cause tooth decay and gum inflammation.

I personally have not used any toothpaste (as it contains too many chemicals) since 1993. I use 3% food-grade hydrogen peroxide in a spray bottle (only use hydrogen peroxide in your mouth if you are free of mercury amalgam fillings as peroxide can interact with mercury). I occasionally use Gum Joy Oil (an anti-inflammatory, cold-pressed oil blend containing mostly hemp and mint oils). I sometimes sprinkle Celtic sea salt on my toothbrush before I brush. Celtic sea salt creates an alkaline environment in the mouth that prevents harmful bacteria from overgrowing. It is beneficial to gargle with Celtic sea salt diluted in water. I also often rub coconut oil directly onto my gums and teeth before I go to bed. Coconut oil's antiseptic qualities destroy bacteria that contribute to tooth decay.

Many people are now opting for the removal of mercury fillings and are replacing them with the more attractive and healthy gold, composite, or porcelain fillings. For two days leading up to the mercury being removed from the body, and for a period of two-to-three weeks after the mercury has been removed, I recommend including in your daily diet as much as 3,000 to 5,000 milligrams of whole-food vitamin C (*camu camu berry powder*), 3 tablespoons of *Sun Is Shining Superfood*, and 5,000 to 10,000 mg of MSM (*mercury bonds with sulfur*). These additional nutrients are taken to protect the body against the damaging effects of mercury vapor emitted during the removal process and to detoxify any mercury residue from the system.

Eyes

Sometimes the beauty of one feature is enough to carry all the others. This seems particularly true with the eyes. On a raw-diet, eye color can, and usually does, change over time. Typically, on a raw-diet, the eyes soften, lighten, become more luminescent, and show more gold, green, or blue.

Dark circles under the eyes are related to having an exhausted adrenal system. Coffee contributes to this, as do other stimulants, such as refined sugar (*soda, candy*), cigarettes, and recreational drugs. Dark circles may also be caused by a potassium overdose (*eating too many foods high in potassium*) such as bananas, dried fruit, avocados, durian, nuts, and sprouts.

Dark circles can be corrected by eating foods high in organic sodium, such as celery, chard, kale, spinach, olives, and unwashed sea vegetables and by using Celtic sea salt.

Cucumbers and pumpkin seeds may also be effective in alleviating this condition.

Puffiness under the eyes is often caused by too much sodium in the body. This causes the body to retain water. To correct this, eat more high-potassium foods, such as bananas, dried fruits, avocados, durian, nuts, and sprouts. Also, remove salt from the diet.

Over 500 million nerve endings arrive in each eye. Nutritionist Bernard Jensen perfected the ancient science of iridology (*the study of the iris*). He demonstrated that the irises accurately reflect the state of the internal organs. The more perfect one's health, the more perfect is the iris. Imperfections, such as spots and irregularities around the pupil, indicate congestion, constipation, candida, or some other condition.

Eye-beauty is a natural by-product of real and deep tissue cleansing caused by eating a raw-food-based diet, colon cleansing, a variety of nutritional cleanses and various forms of fasting. Once one is sufficiently cleansed, fasting brings forth a divine, almost startling, radiance, from the eyes.

Blueberries, bilberries, lychees, and goji berries (*sometimes called wolfberries or lyceum*) are excellent foods for improving eyesight. These foods contain high quantities of antioxidants. In fact, of 40 common fruits and vegetables tested, blueberries tested number one in antioxidants (*as reported by Dr. Prior, director of the USDA studies*).

Correcting poor eyesight is possible by eating raw-plant-foods (*especially those rich in cleansing sulfur compounds such as garlic, onions, and cayenne*), taking in rich antioxidant sources (*to support eye nutrition*), including Sunfood Nutrition's Krill Oil in the diet (*to feed the eye its most important nutrient: docosahexaenoic acid or DHA*), avoiding any and all cooked oils and fats (*these clog the tiny capillaries of the eyes and lead to cataracts*), reading under only full spectrum lights (*reading in the dark causes eye stress*), sufficiently resting the eyes, and emotional cleansing surrounding childhood traumas *(which are often linked to eye stress and poor eyesight).* I also recommend studying books like *Relearning To See* by Thomas Quackenbush, and *Take Off Your Glasses And See* by Dr. Jacob Liberman.

Voice Beauty

Singing is one of our most uplifting natural urges. Through internal cleansing and many years of eating raw-foods, the voice takes on more pleasant tones in both the higher ranges and the deeper baritone ranges.

Avoiding any and all dairy products, which are notorious for forming excess mucus that damages the delicate resonant sinus cavities, is the first step in unleashing vocal beauty.

Fresh pineapple and grapefruit juice are great for vocal cord inflammation. These raw-foods contain bromelain, an anti-inflammatory enzyme.

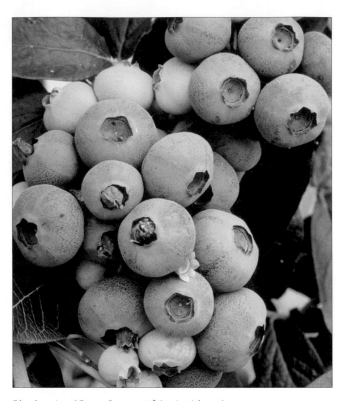

Blueberries *(Great Source of Antioxidants)*

Mint is an excellent vocal tonic. Mint leaves of all types help soothe the voice. Mint contains residual menthol, a relaxing, yet invigorating substance that opens and heals the bronchial tubes, Eustachian tubes, sinuses, and the vocal cords.

Mint is also a great breath freshener.

Mint leaves may be used in cold teas, sun teas, or salads.

Eucalyptus honey contains eucalyptol, which is a substance with properties similar to menthol. Eucalyptol helps to relieve and heal damaged vocal tissue.

Red clover buds contain a nutrient called trifolin. Trifolin acts favorably on the vocal cords. It can be utilized by drinking red clover tea. This tea can be obtained at the local herb shop or natural-food store. Red clover buds may also be eaten fresh and raw with a salad.

Berberin, a natural anti-fungal compound found in blackberries, has an influencing effect on vocal beauty. Berberin is also found in barberry and radishes.

If a sore throat is affecting the voice, chewing on little pieces of ginger, drinking ginger juice, or consuming ginger tea with raw honey will be effective in reducing the inflammation.

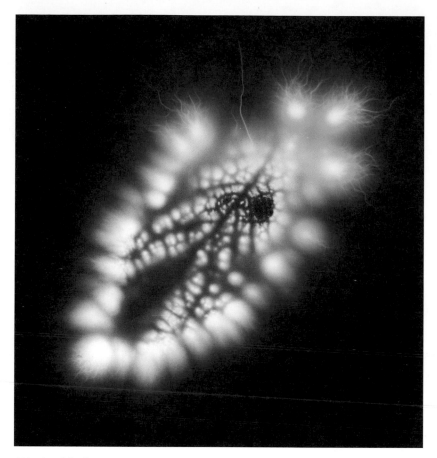

Mint Leaf *(Kirlian Image)*

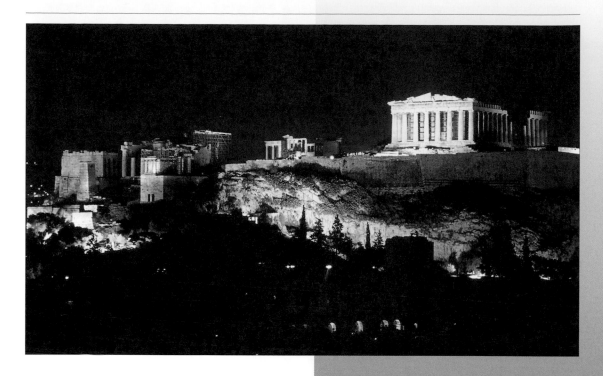

xercise oxygenates and enlivens all the tissues, bringing more charisma and color into the complexion.

Because the buildup of bodily wastes can become increasingly toxic, we need daily exercise so that the bloodstream can move through the muscles forcefully, carrying away these toxic residues.

Although there are many different forms of physical exercise, yoga seems to be the most wonderful balancer for today's fast-paced, high-stress lifestyles.

Exercises generally fit into two distinct categories: those that stretch the muscles and those that strengthen them. Yoga is effective for accomplishing both of these, while adding deep, oxygenating breathing to one's exercise program. Deep breathing, in itself, is a great cleanser that imparts rich-ness to the skin and grace to the physique.

Yoga means "union." Physical types of yoga fall into the classification of Hatha Yoga. In Sanskrit, the word "hatha" is a com-bination of the syllables "ha," the Sun, and "tha," the moon. The mixture and balance of

> *"A Yogi is not so much interested in finding the Fountain of Youth as he/she is in continuing the Spirit of Youth to the very end. There is nothing that will fill the human heart with more cheer than the practice of Yoga."*
>
> *Theos Bernard,*
> *Yoga Gave Me Superior Health*

these two primary forces is the essence of physical yoga.

Considering there are close to 700 muscles in the human body, it would be nice to incorporate each muscle into our exercise program. This is accomplished most completely by practicing various forms of yoga.

Yoga moves energy throughout the body and releases memories, perceptions, and emotions. It also helps the body eliminate the residues of the cooked foods we have eaten over the years that are stored in our calves, thighs, torso, and buttocks, as well as in our arms, back, shoulders, and neck.

Squeezing and twisting your muscles is similar to squeezing and twisting a soiled washcloth; it has a cleansing effect, yet at the same time it opens the tissues to receiving more nourishing fluids. This type of motion is great for the intestines.

Inverted positions (*head stands, shoulder stands*) bring more blood flow and nutrients to the head and scalp. This type of motion is great for the glands, brain, and hair.

Yoga of all kinds is more beneficial if done consistently, and possibly at the same time every day. One will be amazed how the body will accept activity, no matter how challenging, if it is done at the same time each day.

Yoga is infinite. I find that if I get bored with one type of yoga practice, I shift to another and do different poses. There are so many yoga postures that one is well challenged to try them all in a lifetime.

Currently, I personally enjoy a mix of Anusara, Ashtanga, Iyengar, and Kundalini Yoga with other types of yoga mixed in and my own more mellow yoga practice.

Yoga practitioner and raw-foodist Kim Sol and I developed the *Raw Yoga* DVD at Eden Hot Springs. This DVD presents a whole new insight into yoga in light of the new leading-edge concepts of raw-food nutrition.

Beauty Sleep

We have the saying "beauty sleep" in our language for a profound reason. A healthy slumber rests the muscles of your face and body, as well as your nerves and brain. Sleep is the time when we rejuvenate our skin and connective tissue. Beauty sleep is a restorative: a time for recharging the nerves.

There are no tried and true rules of when to sleep. An afternoon siesta may be appropriate for some, not for others. Some say that the hours of sleep before midnight are the most restful.

Generally, raw-food eaters require two hours less sleep than they did when they ate cooked food. I have known some raw-fooders who sleep only three-to-four hours per night. Many people new to raw-foods expect these kinds of results immediately. This expectation is usually unrealistic. When one begins a raw-food program, sleep requirements may remain the same for several months, or even a year. This depends on the internal state of the body and on the energy required to restore good health and digestion.

How much sleep do we need? The answer is "just the right amount." Too much sleep leaves us sleepy all day, too little leaves us exhausted.

One thing we know is that the more we eat, the more sleep we require. A restful beauty sleep results from going to bed with a clear stomach and a clear mind.

How one sleeps affects how refreshed one feels upon waking. Lower back challenges and sciatica (*shooting pain down the back of the hips and legs*) can be created by sleeping on one's stomach on a soft bed, or sleeping on one's side with a twist in the spine. If sleeping on one's side, having both knees bent equally with a pillow between them helps to prevent an injurious spinal twist. When sleeping on one's back, a pillow under the knees will relieve pressure on the lower back.

Bedding should be firm, yet comfortable. I personally have never taken well to soft beds, raised beds, or waterbeds. I like to sleep on a futon on the floor. I feel this gives me excellent back support.

Sufficient air purification, ionization, and ozonation by a state-of-the-art air purifier, as well as a close proximity to oxygen-producing plants and salt lamps, will make for a more restful sleep *(to request information about air purifiers and salt lamps, call 888-729-3663)*. Non-binding pajamas *(or sleeping naked)* and non-binding covers are also helpful.

— Insomnia —

Insomnia may be corrected by doing hard physical work all day to the point of exhaustion. It is also much easier to fall asleep after the release of an orgasm.

The old raw-food "cure" for insomnia is fresh lettuce juice. Lettuce contains soporific compounds and opiates that in the concentration of a juice have a calming, sedative effect.

More recent research into insomnia recommends an increase of tryptophan *(the chemical precursor to the serotonin neurotransmitter that*

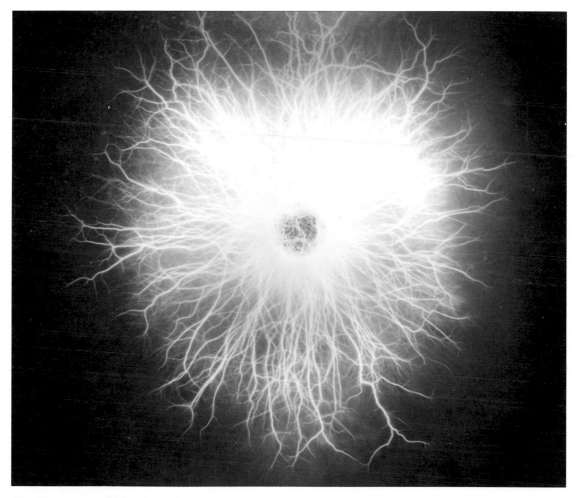

Blue Mangosteen *(Kirlian Image)*

creates euphoric feelings by clearing nerve passages). The common causes of insomnia, such as emotional repression, anxiety, and tension, may be relieved by ingesting tryptophan-rich foods. Tryptophan is found in high protein foods, especially in pumpkins seeds and the durian fruit.

There are no magic pills here. Let us understand that an excellent well-rounded raw-food-based diet along with sufficient exercise brings the body into balance and makes sleeping easy and enjoyable.

Creating regular patterns of relaxing activities before bedtime is an excellent idea. Mild yoga poses, hot baths, meditation, applying beauty masks, and massaging olive oil or coconut oil into your skin are excellent ideas.

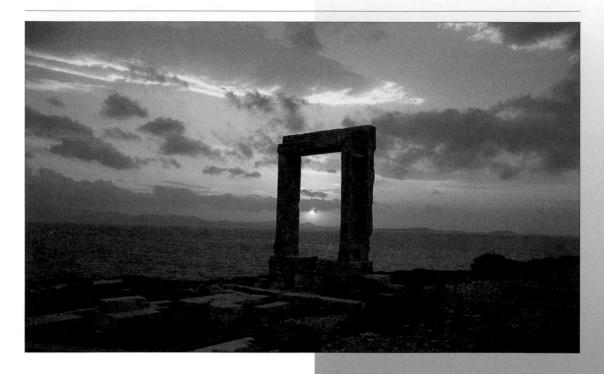

The raw-food lifestyle is startling and transformative. The deeper you allow this information to penetrate your awareness, the more you may realize that the human body is truly a finely-calibrated, animated work of sculpture.

Like any successful health program, this is a dynamic process that employs the trial and success method, step-by-step movement, cleverness, strategy, and fun!

Remember: There are many suggestions in this book and in this lesson chapter. The best idea is to take in the foods and beautifying strategies that you can use and leave the rest for another time. Everything comes in its own time. Enjoy the process. For this beautification process to work, the only thing that matters is that you keep moving forward!

Thinking For Beauty

Sound physical health and beauty begin with a "health and beauty consciousness" produced by a mind that thinks in terms of health and beauty, and not in terms of death, pain, fire, and destruction. This consciousness

LESSON 13:
THE PSYCHOLOGY OF BEAUTY CONSCIOUSNESS

"Cheerfulness and contentment are great beautifiers and are famous preservers of youthful good looks."

Charles Dickens

"The secret of attractiveness is in developing a magnetic personality."

Walter Russell, Artist, Architect, Author, Philosopher

"The human body is the best picture of the human soul."

— *Ludwig Wittgenstein, British Philosopher*

"Beauty of whatever kind, in its supreme development, invariably excites the sensitive soul to tears."

— *Edgar Allen Poe*

"Always remember your true beauty comes from within, no matter what methods you use to beautify your body on the outside. If your heart is filled with envy, hate, jealousy, and ugly, unhappy thoughts, it will discolor your aura for all to see. What you thought yesterday, you will live today. What you think today, you will live tomorrow. If you want to live a life filled with health, beauty, joy, and happiness, then think only of that which is beautiful, and you will be beautiful."

— *Anonymous*

"The secret of beauty in anyone is in having beautiful thoughts which illumine the whole features."

— *Walter Russell,*
Artist, Architect, Author, Philosopher

In your image of yourself is your future self. You live into the picture you hold of yourself. Your body reflects your thoughts exactly.

Everything is an external manifestation of an internal conversation. If you have a beautiful, loving inner nature, your outer world of life and relationships will be marked by prosperity.

Beauty of mind, body, and spirit can only be kept permanently by those individuals who are persistent enough to shut out disharmony, negative thoughts, and confusion. Whatever images the self allows to flash through the screen of the mind are instantaneously stamped upon the flesh of the physical body. True beauty is never fleeting; it remains, because, in the final analysis, it is self-created.

Beauty is holistic. An opening of the mind erases lines in even the most wrinkled complexion. A warming of the heart transforms even the most selfish scrooge. A more generous disposition drops pounds from the heaviest frame. Increased feelings of love and harmony restore the suppleness of youth in the most elderly.

In essence, beautiful individuals become beautiful because they acquire the habit of thinking in terms of beauty. Thoughts of beauty always precede the manifestation of beauty.

Laughter

"From the moment I picked up your book until I laid it down, I was convulsed with laughter. Some day I intend on reading it."

— *Groucho Marx*

"Ridentem dicere verum, quid vetat." (What forbids us to tell the truth while laughing?)

— *Horace*

leads to behaviors such as temperance of habits in eating and properly balanced physical activities.

Thoughts — positive or negative — etch themselves into the face and record themselves in the character of the individual. The power of thought has control over every cell of your body. You are your own sculptor. The habitual presence of high and noble thoughts polishes the face, defines the stature, and builds the countenance. High purpose and genuine enthusiasm create an immaculate beauty. Thoughts alone can overwhelm the influence of clothing and cosmetics.

> "The most wasted of all days is that one in which one has not laughed."
>
> — *Camfront*

> "Humor is better than a tumor."
>
> — *Dr. Jonathan Bailey*

Laughter is nature's greatest beautifier. Laughter is the divine sculptor. Joy is nature's grand cosmetic. Smile and your digestion will improve. Unconditional laughter may be the highest vibration in the universe.

Laughter is an attribute of beauty that the divine forces are constantly pouring into the universe. Mineral-rich, nutrient-dense raw-plant-foods, noble thoughts, and harmonious feelings of love and joy attract more of the cosmic outpourings of laughter into your body — they make it easier for you to laugh and enjoy life!

The world is made young with laughter. A joke a day keeps the doctor away. S/he who laughs, lasts. Laughter is longevity.

I know from my lecturing experience that audiences are more receptive to a message told on the light, funny side. Humor has the power to courteously shift attitudes and perceptions. Humor is a gentle teacher. Share a laugh, and it's likely that you will have created a unique bond with others.

If you have the courage to meet your challenges with cheer, you will keep the sunshine sparkling in your eyes and the smile in your cheeks. When you transmute frustration into fascination and anger into laughter, it means your energy level is much higher than before. It means barriers are breaking down, progress is being made, and you are having more fun.

Laughter

One is not taught in college.
The key to ultimate knowledge:

Laughter —
Charges, enlarges,
Grasps, recreates
At accelerated rates
Renews, redefines
Erases wrinkled lines.

A closer look reveals
Everything is funny!
The future can only be sunny.

Laughter makes the world young.
Laughter speaks a universal tongue.

A winning smile.
Lasts a long, long while.

When life becomes
Fun and laughter
You'll open a new chapter
And sow a seam
In what things mean

Laughter mends chaos and fright
With wisdom, light, and clever insight.
Laughter silences every thought
As it heals everything you've got.

Laughter seeks the highest beat
Can knock a grown man from his feet.
Shifts one's mood
Is better than food.

Laughter is sunshine
In the home.
(Please let's make that known.)

No matter what's done,
If it's done with laughter,
It's bound to live
Happily ever after.

When it's said and done
And the journey's been run
When your time has passed,
Remember:
Only smiles and laughter last.

Once you have awoke
And seen through the smoke
Unlocked the hidden yoke.
You'll get the cosmic joke:

It's a punch line —
All the time!

Flow

"Beauty arises in the stillness of your presence…Beyond the beauty of external forms, there is more here: something that cannot be named, something ineffable, some deep, inner, holy essence. Whenever and wherever there is beauty, this inner essence shines through somehow."

— *Eckhart Tolle, The Power of Now*

The present civilization is one in which the population has spent trillions of dollars on beauty products, while the fundamental art of eating for beauty and thinking for beauty are only now becoming known. A new type of beauty culture awaits all those who eat and think for beauty, because clean, pure thoughts, laughter, and mineral-rich, nutrient-dense, raw-plant-foods become the foundation of all lasting physical and spiritual beauty.

Beautiful food and noble thoughts rebuild the body on their own plan. They extract the true you.

And that is my goal: to bring you more into alignment with your own true pattern of life. That is the direction of perfection. The nearer one is to this divine perfection, the higher the level of beauty that is manifested.

What you are in the end is a feeling. That is what your spirit is — the real you is a feeling

in nature. When your logical mind is switched off, and questioning through intellectual activity halts, then what is left is your spiritual essence. Once you tap into what that essence is, then you will know what your life is about.

When you feel this essence and live by it, you instantly become better at everything you do. You enter into a "flow."

Have you ever been in a flow before, where everything was just perfect? Where you knew you were in a space where only amazing things could happen? It might have been the perfect date. It might have been several hours during a final exam, where everything just flowed. It might have been a fulfilling vacation. It might have been while playing music. I remember one time having an amazing day in high school sports, where I had unbelievable speed and strength, unlike anything I had ever experienced.

I was always fascinated by these moments of "flow." These moments are glimpses of our human potential. I always sought to find a way to get back into the elusive flow.

I discovered, much to my surprise, that through the raw lifestyle, these moments of flow occur much more often and eventually become a way of life. This was a strong confirmation to me that if we keep seeking, we shall find.

It seems that when your body is in tune and every cell is resonating properly, then it is much easier to be in the right place at the right time. When you are in a state of flow synchronicities occur more frequently. Everything becomes more natural. Flow is actually our natural state of being. This is true magic.

Conclusion

In some way, we are all born into a complex lie. We live today in a world of unlimited resources and unlimited wealth — exactly the opposite of what we have been told. We live in a world where alchemistry is real — where lead can be turned into the white powder of gold! The fact that individuals every day create incredible value out of nothing more than an idea — go from rags to riches almost overnight — is proof positive that radical transformation is possible for anyone at any time.

There is no magic pill, but there is a magic process. There is a beautification process we can all undergo through which we can begin to unwind bad habits, old injuries, illnesses, and negative attitudes, and through which we can begin to get a profound new understanding of life.

Mother Nature has given you permission to be beautiful. A tree or a deer never feels guilty about being beautiful. Beauty and grace is our natural state. The fact that you are reading this now is proof that at some deep level you know you deserve something more.

Raw-plant-foods are the most consistent with the physical, mental, spiritual, and idealistic aspirations of the human race. Within the genre of raw-plant-food, all we need is balance — and the wisdom and creativity that arise from that state.

The raw-food lifestyle is really about enjoying every precious moment of life. Raw-food is fun. Fruit is fun. Fresh juices are fun. I invite you to join me in choosing only to do things that are fun.

Eat raw-plant-foods, cleanse your system, receive your beauty sleep, engage in exactly the perfect amount of exercise, and open your mind, and you will become more deeply and profoundly alive.

How alive can you become? What is the depth of your human potential?

With every organ functioning optimally, the human body becomes a thing of grace, joy, and happiness; takes on strength, energy and mental alertness; and becomes a wholesome, clean, strong, healthy system able to physically and spiritually express one's mission on Earth.

"Exuberance is beauty," wrote William Blake. Discover what it is like to move through the world with confidence and an exuberant attitude. Worry, depression, and anxiety show up in slumping shoulders, a collapsed chest, and a downward stare. An exuberant attitude, cheer, happiness, laughter, and wonder cause the shoulders to move back, the chest to expand, and the head to ride high.

Offer beauty in this world. Become fair. Create a dream life. More and more, find yourself in the presence of confident, beautiful individuals who can inspire you.

Cultivate an attitude of gratitude for the splendor of the present moment, and for the abundance that life offers — this is the true foundation of beauty and prosperity. Everything is a blessing in disguise. Take things lightly and you more readily enjoy each moment.

Live in the eternal moment — in the middle of the flow — now. Be raw now. Avoid overly concerning yourself with the future or the past. Tomorrow is a mystery and yesterday is history.

Of little interest now are the merchants of ancient Greece, the generals of the Spartan armies, the kings of Mycenea. But what has and will last forever from the civilization of ancient Greece is its cultural feeling — its immortal feeling of beauty.

Rejuvenate and surpass the ancient beauty ideals. Tap into beauty as an onrushing force throughout all of nature that strives for purer and more pristine perfection. Pursue perfection and know that the slightest effort spent is always remembered.

Enjoy great health, in the fullest meaning of the word. Achieve inner and outer cleanliness. Nourish and create clear, fresh, smooth skin. Allow your eyes to sparkle. Bring a bountiful lustre into your hair. Welcome into your life the practice and symmetry of yoga. Stand with confidence. Walk with rhythm and grace. Nurture a pleasing countenance.

Greet others with charm and vivacity. Breathe deeply. Cultivate a magical laugh. Make every day the best day ever!

This is your scene, your dance, your party, your never-ending birthday bash!

Eden has never been lost! It is right where you are at now.

Look around you. Listen. Feel the vibrations of the deserts, forests, and mountains. The Earth is beautiful. All is well with the world.

Bless you, and may God beautify your journey.

A Gift

May your days be fulfilling,
And your nights be thrilling.

May every venture,
Become an adventure.

May you walk the land,
And play in the sand.

May you sail the oceans,
And drink magical potions.

May you splash and have fun,
Under an endless summer sun.

May you hear the violins
In soft, warm winds.

May you dance to flutes,
And taste exotic fruits.

May your heart overflow,
Everywhere you go.

May your limits be tested,
And your best day be bested.

May your moments of glory,
Be retold in a story.

May your life be blessed,
And good fortune be your guest.

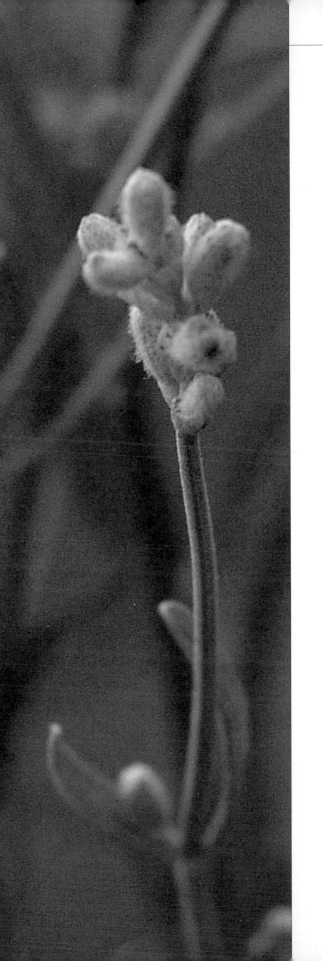

WHAT IS BEAUTY

What is beauty?
Can you tell?
In the radiant flower
And enticing smell?

A spray of blossoms
Enrapturing, capturing,
Splattered with tone and tint,
Sharp, crisp, as menthol in mint.
Ennobled by form, color,
Each unlike another.

On life´s innovative side,
There is a force that strives,
To make everything more alive!
More purity, elegance,
Ambient radiance.

Can you see
In the shape of the bee
That harmony, design, and order
Animates all of Nature?

What is beauty?
Did you feel
That you could strive
For the ideal?

Idealism of character
Is a perfecting factor.
It attracts the commitment,
The grace,
To transform,
Be reborn,
To awe and inspire,
Never to tire,
To make a new start
By becoming a work of art!

To go for it,
More than ever before,
To surpass all your goals
And then go for more.

Beauty is a jewel,
A talisman of renewal,
An infinite wealth,
The essence
Of perfect health.

What is beauty?
Did you discover?
A shift, a lift
In the arms of a lover?

A wink, a stare,
From one so fair.

The delicate touch
Of a partner's grace
At the perfect moment,
In the perfect place.

The beauty essence
Is a magical presence.
It is the highest sensation
And deepest inclination.

The pure glow of refined skin,
A tan physique, long and thin.

Consider the beauty
Of Asian serenity,
African physique,
Exotic, unique,
Nordic hair,
The American stare,
Olive tan,
The Mediterranean man.

What is beauty?
Is it time to unleash
The idealism that was
Ancient Greece?
The search for the Golden Fleece?

Imagine that Beauty
Could launch a thousand ships!
Over a thousand miles
And a thousand trips!

That Beauty
Could pervade the master-works of
Phidias, Praxiteles,
The brilliant philosophy of Thales,
The cleverness of Anaximander,
The brilliance of Alexander.

Shall we revive, recollect
The cosmic architects,
Elegant prefects,
Colossal marble stones,
Hushed spectator tones?

The ancient beauty ideal
Is one we still can feel.
One we can revive
And make even more alive.

What is beauty?
Is it time to see?
Beauty,
Telemetry,
Perfect symmetry.
Charisma,
Chemistry,
The grand mystery!
Biological,
Physiological.
Excellence,
Effervescence.

Mystical mathematics,
Schematics,
Yoga, contortion,
Harmonious proportion.

What is beauty?
Where do we start?
And what of the beauty in art?

Art is clever,
On a canvas or stage.
Art mirrors the spirit of the age.
An interstellar
Truth-teller,
Like a wise-old sage.

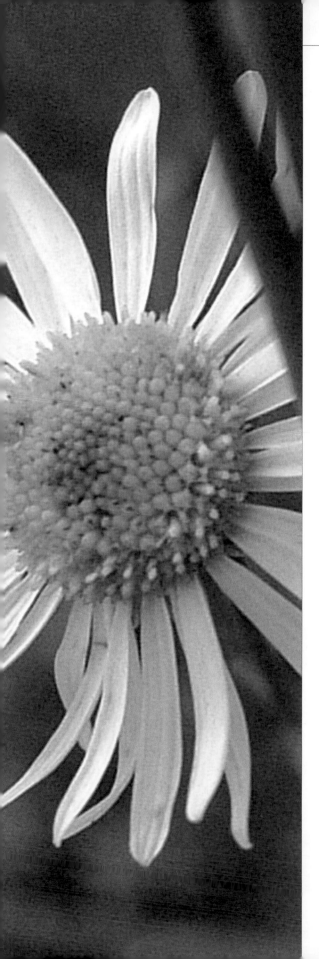

What is beauty?
Did you expect
That everything
Is perfect?

It´s the way we´re designed,
Beauty feeds the mind.

Thoughts of the ideal
Create an energy field.
Forms an attraction
And each proper action.

Beauty peels,
Reveals,
The deep meaning,
Of inner cleaning.

Beauty itself,
Inspires noble deeds,
Spreads the vital fruit seeds,
Laughs...beckons...calls,
Walks through walls,
Strides the hallowed halls,
Overcomes all resistance,
By grace and persistence.

What is beauty?
Could you describe?
Is it possible to become
So much more alive?

The ability to improve and perfect
Arises when you select:
Only thoughts that are grand
In your hourglass of sand.

What is beauty?
In the orchid, the poppy?
The morning dew?
The meadow hue?
Does beauty depend on the point of view?
Or is it the same for me and you?

What is beauty?
What do we know?

Is it inner glow?
Radiant skin?
The will to win?
Abundant vitality,
Recreating reality?

What we find
In short, in kind,
Is that...
Kind words create attractive lips,
A flexible attitude creates
attractive hips,
More sharing creates
a slim physique,
An inner lustre creates hair
that's unique.

Beauty is a spiritual thing
That inspires the bells of heaven
to ring,
Causes the spirits to prance!

To leap and to dance!
To rise from their slumber,
Enticed by form, number.

When one feels:
Cosmic meals,
Atlantean ideals,
The millennial wheels,
Then it is known
And it is shown
That the finest solution
Is an internal, spiritual, revolution.

What is beauty?
Have you known?
The scent of beauty and its charm
Makes one immune from harm.

Beauty brings rewards so great
To completely rewrite your fate.

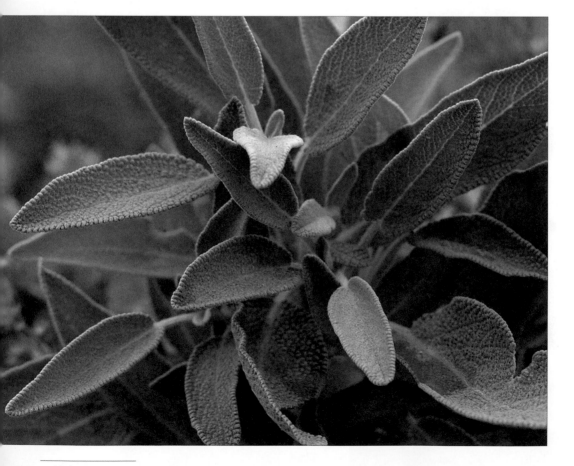

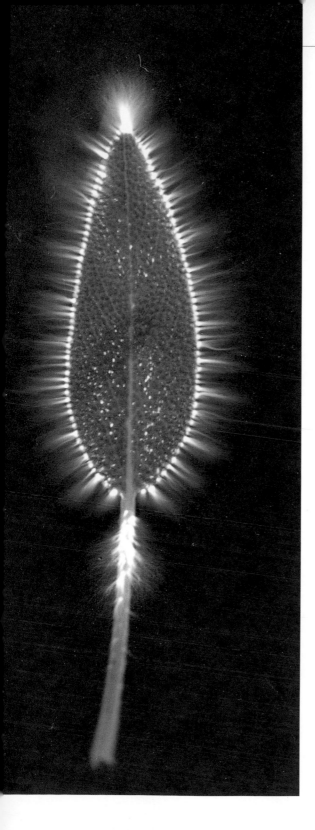

Whatever spell you're living in,
Beauty can take you in,
Balance yang and yin,
Turn a loss to a win,
Make you an angel, on the tip of a pin,
As you sail off, into the din.

May you be blessed
To be better than the best,
To find delight in every sight ,
To enjoy…
All that is congenial, twice,
Everything beautiful, thrice,
Everything ideal, four times or more.
To eat the fruit and plant the core.

And if you're clever,
If you seek and you endeavor,
And notice the way you've been leaning,
You'll discover the meaning:
Beauty is a feeling.

HOT SPRINGS

*A*gamemnon, the leader of the Greek armies during the Trojan War, is said to have brought wounded soldiers to Balcova Hot Springs near Izmir, Turkey. Even today, the Balcova pools are known as "The Baths of Agamemnon."

Hot springs and saunas work to cleanse and beautify the body by stimulating circulation in the muscles and skin, and by increasing internal enzymatic activity.

The skin plays a major role in the eliminative value of hot springs and saunas. We have more than 100 perspiration glands in a single square centimeter of skin! It is through the pores that up to thirty percent of our body wastes are eliminated. This elimination is greatly stimulated by sweating. Perspiring is not only necessary for our health, but it also makes our skin beautiful.

Soaking in salty hot spring waters draws oils, fat-soluble toxic materials, and toxic fats out of the skin. Soaking in sulfurous hot spring waters allows the skin to absorb the beauty mineral *(sulfur)* directly.

Hot spring bathing has been shown to:

1. Improve the skin's suppleness.

2. Aid in the synthesis of collagen and elastin, thus building elastic connective tissue and erasing wrinkles.

3. Be loaded with enzymes which scour, clean, and nourish the skin. *(Natural mud baths are particularly loaded with enzymes. In 1956, F.M. Bilyans'kii of the Russian Institute of Biochemistry discovered that the curative properties of muds could be ascribed to the presence of the enzyme catalase.)*

4. Help to heal acne, eczema, rashes, psoriasis, and other skin challenges.

5. Help to build strong bones and teeth through the minerals that can be absorbed directly into the body through the skin.

Hot Springs Retreats

I conduct many lectures, seminars, and workshops that range from three days to one week at various Hot Springs Retreat Centers around the world. During these workshops, we discuss and apply, with our wonderful guests, the beauty secrets discussed throughout this book.

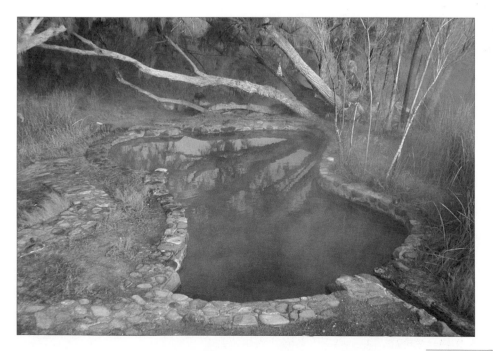

NON-BEAUTIFYING PLANT FOODS

*T*he following are plant foods that I believe disfavor beauty:

Beans

The Pythagoreans, like the Egyptians who preceded them, abstained from eating beans. They held beans to be unclean.

Beans *(legumes)* contain coarse, irritating proteins that cause inflammation.

Beans naturally contain a host of alkaloid toxins. These protect the beans from animals that would eat them in the wild. Several of these compounds are toxic cyanogens, such as cyanide *(found in wild lima beans)*. Raw beans and peas also contain hemagglutins *(causing the blood to clump up)* as well as substances that inhibit the digestion of protein. Raw fava beans are very toxic, containing vicine, covicine, and isouramil. Some individuals cannot break down these toxins at all. These toxins inhibit red blood cells from delivering oxygen to the rest of the body, bringing on headaches, dizziness, nausea, vomiting, severe abdominal pain, and fever. Though these toxins are mostly destroyed by cooking, their presence indicates beans are not a natural food for human consumption.

Raw peanuts would be the best bean to eat. Unfortunately, they are typically contaminated with aflatoxin, a harmful fungus. However, Sunfood Nutrition's Wild Amazonian Peanut is aflatoxin free and remains one of the most interesting food products on the market today.

Soy beans are the least coarse of the beans. They contain more fat, relative to protein. However, soy oils *(e.g. partially hydrogenated soybean oil)* have an anti-thyroid effect that slows down the thyroid, leading to a slower metabolism and weight gain. Eating raw soy beans may enlarge the pancreas as they contain toxins known to be protein uptake inhibitors.

Potatoes

Potatoes are a nightshade family food. The nightshade family of plants contain various

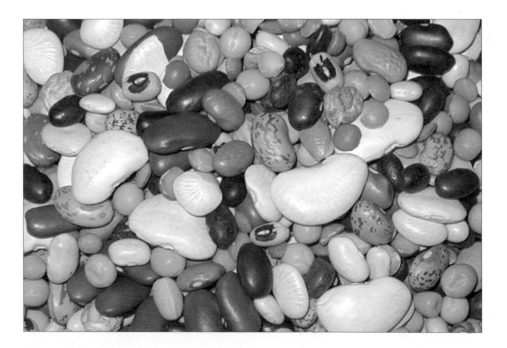

types of toxins. Some nightshade species, such as datura *(jimson weed)*, henbane, and mandrake, may even be deadly if eaten.

Baked potatoes are not only very sugary/starchy and fattening, they also contain the irritating alkaloid toxins solanine and chaconine, which affect the nerves. Solanine is most present in the eyes and sprouted portions of the potato, yet is also found in the skin and throughout the root in lighter concentrations.

Cereal Grains

Many cereal grain seeds *(such as wheat berries)* are so hybridized that they contain too much gluten. Gluten is an irritating inflammatory substance that can actually burn the sensitive lining of the intestines. Products made from wheat seeds *(bread, pasta)* can actually cause our face to become puffy. These products, like other starchy carbohydrates *(baked potato)*, tend to make our skin pale and pasty in appearance.

ℛEFERENCES

There are many documents, books, magazines, websites, and — most importantly — many people, whose insights have enlightened this book. The following list of books is by no means complete, it simply reflects some of the best works that have assisted in the creation of **Eating For Beauty**.

Blatant Raw-Foodist Propaganda by Joe Alexander
  (Blue Dolphin Publishing, Nevada City, California, 1990)

Bonobo, The Forgotten Ape by Frans Lanting and Frans de Waal
  (University of California Press, Los Angeles, 1997)

Children of the Sun by Gordon Kennedy
  (Nivaria Press, Ojai, California, 1998)

Coconut Oil Miracle, The by Bruce Fife
  (Avery Publ., New York, 2004), quoted with permission.

Continuous Creation: A Biological Concept of the Nature of Matter by Wilfred Branfield
  (Happiness Press, Magalia, 1994)

Conscious Eating by Gabriel Cousens, M.D.
  (North Atlantic Books, Berkeley, 2000)

Dark Side of the Brain, The by Harry Oldfield and Roger Coghill
  (Element Books, Dorset, United Kingdom, 1988)

Detox Your World by Shazzie
  (United Kingdom, 2003)

Doctor Jensen's Guide To Body Chemistry & Nutrition by Dr. Bernard Jensen
  (Keats Publishing, Los Angeles, 2000)

Doctor Heinerman's Encyclopedia of Nature's Vitamins & Minerals by John Heinerman
  (Prentice Hall Press, New Jersey, 1998)

Drugs Masquerading As Food by Suzar
  (A-Kar Productions, Oak View, California, 1999)

Fats That Heal, Fats That Kill by Udo Erasmus
  (Alive Books, Canada, 1993)

Feel Good Food by Karen Knowler and Susie Miller
  (Women's Press, UK, 2000)

Free Radicals and Food Additives by P. Addis, P. and G. Warner
  (Taylor and Francis, London, 1991)

From PMS To Menopause by Raymond Peat
  (Eugene, 1997)

Generative Energy by Raymond Peat
  (Eugene, 1994)

Healing Power of Minerals, The by Paul Bergner
  (Prima Publishing, Rocklin, California, 1997)

Healing Power of Papaya by Barbara Simonsohn
  (Lotus Press, Twin Lakes, Wisconsin, 2000)

Healing Power of Plants, The by Frank J. Lipp

Healing with Herbal Juices by Siegfried Gursche
  (Alive Books, Vancouver, 1996)

Heinerman's Encyclopedia of Healing Juices by John Heinerman
  (Reward Books, New Jersey, 1994)

Hemp: What The World Needs Now by John McCabe
  (Sunfood Publishing, San Diego, 2007)

Herbs and Spices by John Heinerman
(Prentice-Hall Parker Publishing Company, Paramus, NJ, 1996)

Hooked on Raw by Rhio
(Beso Entertainment, New York, 2000)

Living in the Raw by Rose Lee Calabro
(Rose Publishing, Santa Cruz, California, 1998)

Miracle of MSM: The Natural Solution For Pain
by Dr. Stanley Jacob, Dr. Ronald Lawrence, Dr. Martin Zucker
(Penguin Putnam, New York, 1999)

Mucusless Diet Healing System, The by Arnold Ehret
(Ehret Literature Publishing Co., Yonkers, NY, 1953 edition)

Naked Chocolate by David Wolfe and Shazzie
(Sunfood Publishing, San Diego, California, 2005)

Naturally Beautiful by Dawn Gallagher
(Universe Publishing, New York, 1999)

Nutrition For Women by Raymond Peat
(Eugene, 1993)

RAW by Roxanne Klein and Charlie Trotter
(Ten Speed Press, Berkeley, California, 2003)

Raw: The Uncook Book by Juliano
(Harper Collins, New York, 1999)

Raw Power! *(2nd Edition)* by Stephen Arlin
(Maul Brothers, San Diego, California, 2000)

Raw Transformation by Wendy Rudell
(North Atlantic Books, Berkeley, California, 2006)

Rawvolution by Matt Amsden
(Harper Collins, New York, 2006)

Spiritual Nutrition by Dr. Gabriel Cousens
(North Atlantic Books, Berkeley, 2005)

Sunfood Diet Success System, The *(6th Edition)* by David Wolfe
(Sunfood Publishing, San Diego, California, 2006)

Sunfood Living by John McCabe
(Sunfood Publishing, San Diego, California, 2007)

Sunlight by Zane R. Kime
(World Health Publications, Penryn, California, 1980)

Survival Into The 21st Century by Viktoras Kulvinskas
(21st Century Publications, 1975)

Ten Essential Herbs by Lalitha Thomas
(Hohm Press, Prescott, Arizona, 1996)

Vitamin C and the Common Cold by Linus Pauling
(Bantam Books, New York, 1970)

Whole Foods Companion by Dianne Onstad
(Chelsea Green, Vermont, 1996)

Wrinkle Cure, The by Nicholas Perricone, M.D.
(Rodale Books, 2000)

Yoga Gave Me Superior Health by Theos Bernard
(Essence of Health, South Africa, 1940)

Your Body's Many Cries For Water by F. Batmanghelidj, M.D.
(Global Health Solutions, Inc., Falls Church, VA, 1997)

ABOUT *K*IRLIAN PHOTOGRAPHY

Kirlian photographic analysis combines high voltage, high frequency, electrical fields, and photographic techniques to make visible subtle energy fields interacting around living and non-living objects of study. These techniques utilize 50,000 volts and a broad range of frequencies to resonate with the test objects, capturing their patterns for analysis.

Christopher Wodtke, Aerospace Engineer, Electrical Engineer, Holographer, and Kirlian Researcher (www.kirlian.com) has, for the last 10 years, been utilizing Kirlian analysis to make subtle energies around us visible. Christopher photographed the Kirlian photos that are brilliantly displayed throughout *Eating for Beauty*.

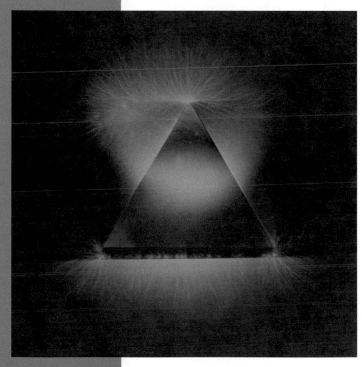

Pyramid *(Kirlian Image)*

Christopher's Kirlian photographs reveal amazing insights into unseen energy fields.

Pyramid energy has been shown to concentrate in the King's Chamber area, revealing the "energy machine" nature of the Great Pyramids.

"Medical Kirlian research will become the Iridology of the future," says Christopher. People with illnesses show major "gaps" in their energy fields, which actually fill back in during their healing process. A major "marker" of diabetes has been discovered, from mass screenings using Kirlian analysis.

Under a "Coor's Foundation" medical grant for research into Gulf War Syndrome, Kirlian analysis was used to monitor patient's progress of healing. Christopher said of the results: "It's repeatable, and a unique way to monitor the individual's healing process." Christopher and his associates have developed a Kirlian diagnostic machine, now in prototyping, that shows the state of one's current health, virtually instantly, using a new type of bio-electrical kinesiology — Kirlian kinesiology. This enables us new insight into the body's workings and into the interactions of our biological structures with medicines, meditations, and magnetic and electrical therapies. Christopher says: "We can see the heartbeat race across the hand with live Kirlian video analysis."

Kirlian.com was selected to help with crop circle analyses. "We are waiting to get samples from some of the new crop circles," says Christopher. Christopher and his associates have developed a "full-stalk" Kirlian camera to show the subtle energies around the bent or changed crops, correlating with reports of "electrical crackling" sounds surrounding recent circles.

The most interesting facet of Kirlian research is Christopher's work with the Shroud of Turin, covered in depth in his forthcoming book: *Kirlian Shroud — In Search of the Face of Christ*. This book documents the newly validated Kirlian Shroud Theory, presented to over 75 countries at The World Foundation for Natural Science's Fifth Congress: New Scientific Outlook at Interlaken, Switzerland, in 1998.

For more information, please visit
www.kirlian.com
or e-mail: kirlian@kirlian.com

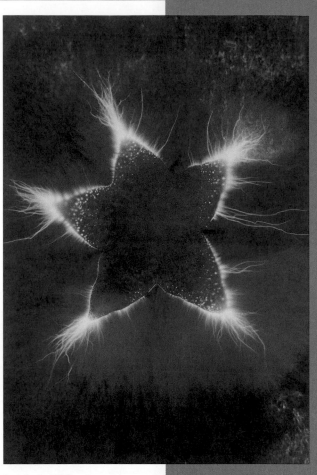

Starfruit *(Kirlian Image)*

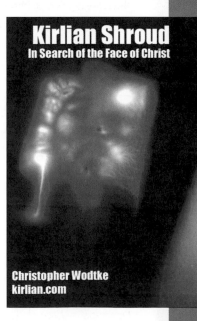

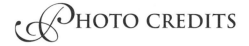

PHOTO CREDITS

All Kirlian Photos by Christopher Wodtke (www.kirlian.com) except for "Raw vs. Cooked Cabbage" from *The Dark Side of the Brain* by Oldfield and Coghill

Acid/Alkaline Chart by Zak Shuman

Front Cover Photo of Rainbeau Mars
(www.rainbeaumars.com)

Introduction Photo by Nick Wellman
(nwellman@bigpond.com)

Cosmic Beauty Photo by Andrew Watson
(andrew_watson@austar.com.au)

Beauty Nutrition Photo by Nick Wellman
(nwellman@bigpond.com)

The Acid/Alkaline Balance Simplified Photo by Glenda Kapsalis
(www.glendakapsalis.com)

The Three Food Classes Photo by Nick Wellman
(nwellman@bigpond.com)

Elements of The Beauty Diet® Photo by Nick Wellman
(nwellman@bigpond.com)

Detoxification & Transformation Photo by Glenda Kapsalis
(www.glendakapsalis.com)

Alchemical Beauty Secrets (The Beauty Minerals) Photo
by Glenda Kapsalis
(www.glendakapsalis.com)

Radish by www.stockfood.com

Beautifying Foods Photo by Graham Tween

Aloe Vera by Glenda Kapsalis
(www.glendakapsalis.com)

Burdock Root by Glenda Kapsalis
(www.glendakapsalis.com)

Coconut Palm by Glenda Kapsalis
(www.glendakapsalis.com)

Cucumbers by www.stockfood.com

Figs by www.stockfood.com

Hemp Seeds by Glenda Kapsalis
(www.glendakapsalis.com)

Macadamia Nuts by www.stockfood.com

Olive by www.stockfood.com

Olive Tree by www.stockfood.com

Onions by Glenda Kapsalis
(www.glendakapsalis.com)

Papayas by Glenda Kapsalis
(www.glendakapsalis.com)

Pumpkin Seeds by www.stockfood.com

Radishes by Glenda Kapsalis
(www.glendakapsalis.com)

Turmeric by www.stockfood.com

Watercress by Glenda Kapsalis
(www.glendakapsalis.com)

The Beauty Diet® Photo by Graham Tween

Mint by Glenda Kapsalis
(www.glendakapsalis.com)

Body Beauty (Skin, Hair, Nails, Teeth, Eyes, Voice) Photo
by Kylie Hood
(kyliehood@hotmail.com)

Blueberries Photo by www.stockfood.com

Yoga & Beauty Sleep Photo by Terrance Klassen
(Top Stock Images)

The Psychology of Beauty Consciousness by Nick Wellman
(nwellman@bigpond.com)

Appendix A: Hot Springs Photo by Carl Barna

Appendix B: Non-Beautifying Plant Foods Photo by Carl Barna

SPECIAL THANKS TO:
Glenda Kapsalis
(www.glendakapsalis.com)

Carl Barna

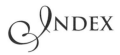

INDEX

arugula 19, 21, 36, 40, 65, 68-69, 72, 74-76, 101, 107, 118-120, 123-124

ascorbic acid 45

Ashtanga Yoga 138

Asian markets 31, 78, 85, 123

aspirin 74

assimilate 2, 51, 61, 68-69

asthma 20

Athens 6, 93-94

atherosclerosis 65, 99

Atlanteans 127

Atlantis 77

ATP 37

avocado 14, 30, 35-37, 50, 57, 68-69, 76, 98, 101, 108, 110-111, 117, 119-121, 123, 124, 129, 132, 133

Ayurvedic medicine 76, 106

B

B vitamins 19, 38, 53-54, 58, 102, 131

bacteria 32, 45, 53-54, 67, 76, 79, 94, 98, 114, 128, 131-133

Bailey, Jonathan 143

baked potatoes 18, 37, 57-58, 114, 132, 156

bananas 30, 122, 133

barium 88

barley seeds 37

barrel cactus 29

basil 119-120, 123

Batmanghelidj, Dr. 44, 158

beans 28, 37, 40, 71, 87, 110, 155, 183-184

Beautifying Foods 12, 73-108, 115, 128, 131

Beauty Beverage 120

Beauty Diet, The 2, 10, 12, 43, 50-51, 66, 109, 115, 131, 177

Beauty Enzymes 52, 58, 113, 184

Beauty Nutrition 11-24

Beauty Products 144, 183-185

Beauty Recipes 110-112, 118-124

Beauty Sleep 1, 137-138, 145

bee pollen 21, 31, 40, 68, 87, 183

beef 21, 32, 36

beer 58, 114

beet 37-38, 72

bell pepper 29, 64, 110-111, 118-120, 123-124

berberin 134

berries 14, 21, 29-30, 39-40, 50, 55, 66, 71, 110, 112-113, 118, 121-122, 124, 130, 132-134, 156, 183-184

best day ever 146, 181-182

beta-carotene 19, 45, 75, 111

betaine hydrochloride 48

bilberries 113

bile acids 68

bile ducts 105

bile flow 76, 105

Biological Transmutations 62-63, 65, 72, 113

biotin 66

Bilyans'kii, F.M. 153

black radishes 105, 118, 124

black walnut hull 52

blackberries 29, 71, 134

bladder 79, 82, 99

Blatant Raw Foodist Propaganda 157

bleaches 23

blender 118, 124

bloating 45, 82

blood purification 92, 106

blood sugar 18, 38, 58, 66, 69, 80

bloodstream 18, 32, 36, 50, 126, 132, 137

Blue Mangosteen 112, 139, 184

blueberries 29, 122, 133-134

blue-green algae 21, 40, 68

body odor 31, 36, 54, 56

bone 59, 62-63, 65-66, 70-71, 84, 87-88, 113, 128-130, 132, 153

bone marrow 22, 32

bone maturation 70

borage seed oil 36-37, 129

bowel irregularities 52, 56-57

BPH (benign prostatic hypertrophy) 103

brain 7, 19, 40, 66-67, 71, 81, 84, 88, 103, 138

brain chemistry 103

Branfield, Wilfred 63, 157

bread 18, 31, 37, 39, 50, 57-58, 105, 110-112, 114, 122, 132, 156

breadfruit 29, 39

breast cancer 22, 75, 96, 101, 129

British Journal of Urology 103

broccoli 10, 19, 21, 50, 65, 68, 76, 112, 123-124

bromelain 58, 134

bronchitis 134

Browning reaction 38

brussel sprouts 21, 68

buckwheat sprout 41

Bunsen burner 17

burdock root 31, 64, 69, 71, 76-77, 92, 119-120

burns 31, 66, 70, 74, 98, 102, 130

butter 20, 37, 79, 81-83, 103, 110, 115, 122, 128, 184

C

cabbage 16, 26, 40, 68

cacao 30, 39, 128, 183

cacao beans 71, 110, 121, 183

cacao butter 115, 128, 184

cacao nibs 71, 110, 121, 183

cadmium 32

Calabro, Rose Lee 158

calcium 25-27, 31-32, 38, 44-45, 62-64, 76, 85, 88, 94, 104, 107, 113

calimyrna figs 86, 120-121, 183

Camfront 143

camu camu 66, 112, 132-133, 184

cancer 20-22, 49, 55, 75-76, 80, 96, 99, 101-102, 106, 129

candida 18, 37, 40, 45-46, 53, 80, 115, 129, 131, 133, 184

candida cleanse 115, 184

canola oil 20, 81-82, 96

cantaloupe 19, 29, 111

capelin 21, 111-112

caprylic acid 79

carbohydrates 18, 32, 35, 37-39, 45, 58, 90, 105, 115, 119, 132, 156

carbon 40, 62, 69, 79

carbonic acid 33

cardiovascular system 19, 110

Carnegie, Andrew 11, 109

carnivores 13, 52

carob 29

carpaine 101

carrots 19, 31, 38, 58, 76, 112

Carthaginians 6

cartilage 63, 66-67, 71

cashews 70, 117, 122-124, 183

catabolic 57

catalase 153

cauliflower 68-69, 112

cavities 48, 63, 65, 134

celery 50, 69, 111-112, 118, 123-124, 132-133

celery juice 47, 77, 82-83

cell growth 69

cell permeability 66

cell repair 69

cells 3, 14, 17, 20, 23, 40, 53-54, 66, 69, 71, 73, 80, 99, 107, 126, 128-130, 155

cellulite 58, 115, 121

Celtic Grey Mineral Sea Salt 44, 47, 111, 118, 120-124, 132-133, 183-184

chaconine 31, 156

Champion juicer 122

chaparral 66, 110, 112-113, 183

chapped lips 38

chard 47, 69, 71, 133

charging water 44

cherimoya 30, 39

cherries 29, 71

chicken 19, 23, 32, 36, 62

Chinese 97, 113, 123-124, 127, 130

chlorella 21, 40

chlorine 26, 44, 62

chlorophyll 28, 31, 33, 50, 71, 78, 83, 88, 92, 110

cholesterol 20, 79-80, 90, 101

chromium 38, 88, 119

chronic fatigue syndrome 45

cigarette smoke 20, 29, 33, 126, 133

cilantro 111, 120

Cinderella 102

cinnamon 119

circulation 80, 106-107, 130, 153

citrus 29, 39, 48, 58, 121

clay 128

cloves 52, 72, 122-124

clutter 57

cocaine 29, 33

coconut butter 37, 77-82, 115

coconut oil 2-3, 20, 36-37, 49, 58, 77-82, 96, 110-112, 114-116, 120, 122, 124, 126, 128-129, 132-133, 140, 183-184

Coconut Oil Miracle, The 81-82, 157

coconut water 31, 39, 45, 77-82, 113-114, 121-123

D

dong quai (*angelica root*) 113

dopamine 40

dragonfruit 29, 39

dried figs 38, 85, 119

drowsiness 70

drugs 23, 29, 33, 38, 53, 81, 88, 103, 106, 114, 133

Drugs Masquerading As Food 157

dry brushing 128

duck 32

dulse 69, 71-72, 120, 122

durian 21, 30, 35-37, 83-85, 103, 111, 133, 140

E

E3 Live 40, 68

Eating For Beauty 3, 17, 22-23, 144

ecstasy 33, 103

eczema 67, 76, 92, 107, 126, 129, 153

edestin 40, 87

eggs 32, 62

Egyptians 82, 97-98, 127, 155

Ehret, Arnold 85, 94, 105, 158

Einstein, Albert 16

EJUVA 52, 115, 184

elastin 63, 153

electrolyte 25, 63, 66, 78

electromagnetic foods 7, 10, 16

electromagnetic radiation 7, 10, 16

electromagnetism 7, 109

Elements of the Beauty Diet 44-54

eliminate 2, 38-39, 51, 58, 67, 69, 99, 114, 126, 132, 138, 153

emotional cleansing 57, 133

emotional fluctuations 56

Emoto, Dr. Masuru 44

endocrine 107

enzyme inhibitors 31-32, 89, 103, 112

enzyme reserves 14-15

enzyme supplements 52

enzymes 52, 54, 57-58, 62, 69-70, 72, 79, 92, 101, 113-114, 119, 153, 184

epidermis 126, 129

Erasmus, Udo 19, 21, 157

erepsin 15, 83

Erotic Cream 121

esoteric 58

Essenes 21, 74

eucalyptus honey 134

eucalyptol 134

euphoria 103

eustachian tubes 134

exercise 6, 37, 45, 51, 57, 63, 67, 93, 115, 137-138, 140, 145

eyes 2, 5, 16, 64, 66, 70, 80-81, 87, 100-101, 107, 115, 125-126, 133-134, 143, 145, 156

F

facial hair 131

facial puffiness 3, 32, 73

faith 33, 58, 109

fasting 6, 43, 53, 56-57, 126, 133

fatigue 15, 45, 71, 80

fats 80-82, 84, 90, 99, 101, 115, 119, 126, 129, 133, 153

Fats That Heal, Fats That Kill 19, 21, 157

fat-soluble 19, 36, 81, 153

fatty acids 19-20, 79-82, 87-88, 90, 95-96, 102, 117, 128-129, 131

fear 33, 55

feijoa 121

fennel 119, 123

fertility 69, 82

fiber 2, 31, 45, 77-79, 87, 99, 101, 120, 128

Fife, Bruce 81-82, 157

fig trees 85

figs 29-30, 38-39, 55, 85-86, 94, 110-111, 115, 119-121, 183

fish 13, 21-23, 32, 51-52, 57, 80, 111-112, 132

Flaminus, T. Quintius 6

flavonol 110

flax oil 10, 20, 37, 88

flax seeds 21, 36-37, 80, 88

flax-seed oil 36, 80, 88

flexibility 63, 66-67, 99

Flight of Daedalus 56

Flora's Premium Vegetal Silica 65, 184

flowers 27, 31, 68, 75-76, 83, 87, 89, 108

fluoride 44

folic acid 45, 99, 105

food combining 50-51, 53, 110

Food Combining Made Easy 51

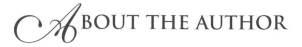

David Wolfe (b. August 6, 1970): David "Avocado" Wolfe is the author of the best-selling books *The Sunfood Diet Success System* and *Naked Chocolate*. He is considered by peers to be the world's leading authority on raw-food nutrition.

David is the middle son of two medical doctors and has an extensive educational background, which gives him a unique perspective in the health field.

David has degrees in Mechanical and Environmental Engineering and in Political Science. He has studied at many institutions, including Oxford University. He concluded his formal education by receiving a Juris Doctor in Law from the University of San Diego.

David conducts 70 to 80 health lectures and seminars each year in the United States, Canada, Europe, and the South Pacific. He hosts at least 5 health, healing, and beauty retreats each year at various retreat centers around the world. You may view his current schedule at: www.sunfood.com/events.html

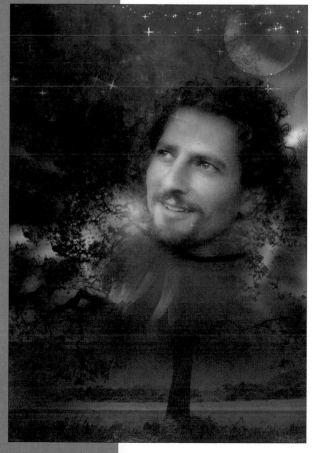

David "Avocado" Wolfe

In addition to his action-packed lecture schedule, David is currently completing several new books and playing the drums in his all-raw rock and roll group — The Healing Waters Band.

Other than a passion for raw-food nutrition and music, David's favorite hobbies include: hiking, yoga, nature adventures, surfing, writing poetry, and spending time with loved ones.

To book David Wolfe on a television or radio show, for an interview, or a seminar please contact:

Sunfood Nutrition, Inc.
Phone: 888-RAW-FOOD
(888-729-3663)
Fax: 619-596-7997
International: +001-619-596-7979
E-mail: nature@sunfood.com
Websites: www.sunfood.com
www.davidwolfe.com

THE FRUIT TREE PLANTING FOUNDATION

www.fruittreefoundation.org

"Nothing in the world gives me more satisfaction than planting fruit trees. As I have always chosen to channel my energy and finances into environmentally-friendly, sustainable, and healthy directions, I founded the nonprofit Fruit Tree Planting Foundation as a place where we could all vote with our money for a better, happier, more abundant, forested future on Earth. Please read about our foundation and decide that you want to donate your time, energy, and/or money to this worthy cause."

— David Wolfe, JD

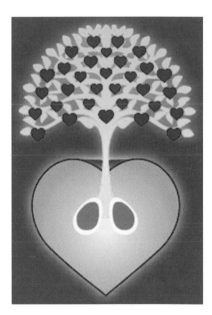

The Fruit Tree Planting Foundation (FTPF) is a unique nonprofit charity dedicated to planting edible, fruitful trees and plants to benefit needy populations and improve the surrounding air, soil, and water.

Our programs strategically plant orchards where the harvest will best serve the community for decades to follow. FTPF plants at places such as homeless shelters, drug rehab centers, low-income areas, international hunger relief sites, and animal sanctuaries. FTPF's projects benefit the environment, human health and animal welfare — all at once!

FTPF's goal is straightforward: to collectively plant 18 billion fruit trees for a healthy planet (approximately 3 for every person alive). Fruit trees heal the environment by cleaning the air, improving soil quality, preventing erosion, creating animal habitat, sustaining valuable water sources, and providing healthy nutrition.

We envision a place where one can have a summer picnic under the shade of a fruit tree, breathe the clean air it generates, listen to the songbirds it attracts, and not have to bring anything other than an appetite for the healthy fruits growing overhead. A world where one can take a walk in the park during a lunch break, pick and eat a variety of delicious fruits, plant the seeds so others can eventually do the same, and provide an alternative to buying environmentally-destructive, illness-causing, chemical-laden products.

FTPF has planted thousands of fruit trees all over the world and provided advice and training for others to do so as well. We have launched a series of exciting new programs and we need your help!

Your tax-deductible charitable investment will help us realize our dream of a sustainable planet for generations to come. As you find you are interested in donating, please send a check or money order payable to:

The Fruit Tree Planting Foundation
P.O. Box 900113
San Diego, CA 92190
USA
www.ftpf.org
info@ftpf.org
Telephone: 831-621-8096
Toll-free: 877-884-7570
Fax: 831-621-7978

While we will be sending you a receipt for your donation, you may want to make a note of this transaction for tax purposes. Thanks for taking action on this important issue.

$\mathcal{D}$AVID WOLFE'S PEAK PERFORMANCE ARCHIVES

www.thebestdayever.com

(Warning! The contents of this website may cause you to have The Best Day Ever!)

A special message from David Wolfe

I have so many tapes of my past lectures, so many notes I have taken over the years, so many great health and success secrets, so many incredible bits of information, that my office and I are overloaded. I literally spent a couple years wondering what to do with all this great stuff! Should I put it into more books? More DVDs? More audio recordings? This stuff is not doing the planet any good sitting here in my office! Then I met a man who recommended that we start a subscription website. We did! We took my material and combined it with information and seminars by the leading women and men in the nutrition and peak performance field. Now all this material is online at thebestdayever.com, and I am so excited!

On this one website you will have access to a literally priceless amount of the most valuable, peak-performance nutritional seminars, documents, interviews, product reviews, and videos ever assembled in one place, at one time!

www.thebestdayever.com demonstrates how to:

- Shed those stubborn, unwanted pounds.
- Experience up-to-date information from America's foremost raw lifestyle authorities *(both women and men)*.
- Leap ahead of the curve in the health and peak performance field.
- Achieve an extraordinary level of energy.
- Radically rejuvenate yourself physically, emotionally, and spiritually.
- Achieve a remarkable level of sensuality, charisma, and sex appeal.
- Enjoy every second of life and really experience The Best Day Ever!
- Explode your creativity.
- Sleep 2–4 fewer hours each night and wake up feeling better than ever!
- Add years (if not decades) to your lifespan.
- Take immediate advantage of secret, yet crucial diet information.

This incredible website gives you complete ACCESS to my text, audio, and video library containing dozens of lectures and CONFIDENTIAL files on nutrition, health, minerals, rejuvenation programs, and exotic information, including information on how to heal some of the most stubborn conditions known to humanity.

Also, the website includes professional nutrition coaching forums where you can get up-to-the-moment answers to your questions. You will also hear live interviews with me on a monthly basis, where I answer your questions and bring you up to date on the latest and greatest. Also, if you are interested, you can tap into my monthly diary blog.

I am a BIG believer in saturating oneself with positive, empowering information. www.thebestdayever.com has been designed to literally bombard you with inspirational text, audio, and video. Much of the material on the site you can download directly onto your computer or iPod and use whenever you want!

www.thebestdayever.com is essentially my uncensored online magazine that allows you to instantly access the latest, most fascinating information in the field. No more waiting by the mailbox. All I do, all day, every day is pursue and live the cutting edge of health, beauty, nutrition, peak performance, vegetarian diets and especially raw-food diets. This information allows you to leap miles ahead of the curve and create astounding rejuvenation and healing now without having to make the same mistakes tens of thousands of others have made.

Why am I doing this? Because the information that is in my brain and computer is expanding far faster than I can publish it in books. I have been perplexed as to what to do with it all. Eventually, the answer appeared: create an online magazine for you! This site was created to give you immediate access to leading edge information to help you instantly enhance the quality of your life.

This is the first time in the history of my career as a peak-performance consultant that I've packaged together so many compelling, life-changing programs into one jam-packed website. Nothing like this website is available on the Internet. This is truly a one-of-a-kind phenomenon. The future is now!

www.thebestdayever.com is constantly updated. This is an ever-growing resource for you and your whole family to enjoy.

If you are inspired to achieve an exceptional state of health, success, beauty, fitness, awareness, joy, sensuality, accomplishment, peak performance, and (most important) fun, then these Peak-Performance Archives are for you!

Check it out and HAVE THE BEST DAY EVER!!!

www.thebestdayever.com

*B*EAUTY PRODUCTS

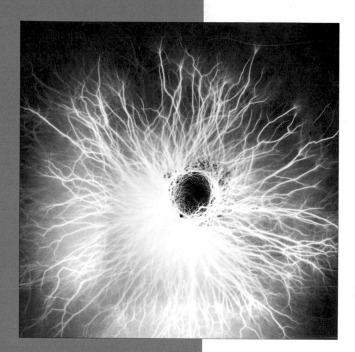

Recommended by David Wolfe
Distributed by Sunfood Nutrition
www.sunfood.com
888-729-3663

BOOKS
Amazing Grace
by David Wolfe and Nick Good
Eating For Beauty by David Wolfe
The Sunfood Diet Success System
by David Wolfe
Sunfood Living by John McCabe
(companion to The Sunfood Diet)
Hemp: What the World Needs Now
by John McCabe
Naked Chocolate
by David Wolfe and Shazzie
Recipes For Beauty by Katie Spiers

RAW-FOOD RECIPE BOOKS
Raw Transformation by Wendy Rudell
Rawvolution by Matt Amsden
RAW by Roxanne Klein
RAW: The Uncook Book by Juliano

FOODS
Sun Is Shining Superfood powder
Agave Cactus Nectar *(raw sweetener) (dark and light)*
Aloe Vera *(fresh)*
Bee Pollen *(100% organic plant protein)*
Black Botija/Botilla Olives
Black Tahini *(raw, organic)*
Cacao Beans *(raw chocolate)*
Cacao Nibs *(raw chocolate)*
Cacao Powder *(#1 in antioxidants)*
Cashew Nuts
(truly raw, out-of-shell)
Cassia *(pod-fruit laxative)*
Celtic Sea Salt
Chaparral *(fresh herb)*
Coconut Oil *(all sizes)*
Figs, dried *(Mission)*
Figs, dried *(Calimyrna)*
Goji Berries
Greek Olives *(sun-dried)*
Hemp Seeds *(raw)*
Hemp Protein *(raw, organic)*
Himalayan Pink Salt

Honey *(Manuka, Organic, Active 10+)*
Italian Olives *(water-cured, in Celtic Sea Salt)*
Kalamata *(Raw Power!)* Olives
Macadamia Nuts *(in shell)*
Maca *(superfood from the Andes)*
Manzanilla Green Olives
  (free of lye, only available part of the year)
Moroccan Olives *(water-cured, in Celtic Sea Salt)*
Olive Oil *(stone-crushed)*
Peruvian Olives *(sun-dried, organic)*
Pumpkin-Seed Butter *(raw)*
Pure Synergy superfood powder
Sacred Chocolate *(high-end, gourmet chocolate bars)*
Schizandra Berries
Vanilla Beans *(raw, organic)*

SUPPLEMENTS
Angstrom-sized Zinc
Angstrom-sized Manganese
Blue Mangosteen Antioxidants
Beauty Enzymes
Camu Camu Berry powder *(Vitamin C)*
Flora's Premium Vegetal Silica *(capsules)*
MSM Powder
Orgono *(Living Silica)*
Pregnenolone *(capsules)*
Pure Radiance C *(whole-food vitamin C source)*
Sunfood Nutrition Krill Oil
Sunfood Nutrition Ormus Gold
Tocotrienols *(High Potency Vitamin E)*

CLEANSING AND WEIGHT LOSS SYSTEMS
EJUVA Herbal Cleanse *(one month)*
EJUVA Parasite Cleanse
EJUVA Candida Cleanse

BODY CARE
Gum Joy Oil *(teeth & gums)*
MSM Lotion *(various scents)*
Cacao Butter *(from Ecuador)*
Coconut Oil *(all sizes)*
Olive Oil *(stone-crushed)*

HAIR CARE
For Normal to Dry Hair:
  Sea Essence Shampoo
  Diamond Crystal Mist Conditioner
For Normal to Oily Hair:
  Earth Essence Shampoo
  Diamond Crystal Mist Conditioner
For Hair Loss or Hair Thinning:
  Apple Cider Vinegar Shampoo
  Pine Shale Shampoo
  EURO Organic Oil

MISCELLANEOUS
Hydrogen Peroxide *(3% food grade)* in a spray bottle

YOGA
Raw Yoga *(DVD)* with Kim Toledo and David Wolfe
Avalon Clothing hemp line *(pants and shirts suitable for yoga)*

* These Beauty Products are currently available from:
www.sunfood.com

Find yourself now
with muscles firm, strong

Living a life that is healthy,
wealthy, and long

Reliving your best years,
regaining your prime

Unencumbered by the winds
of measuring time

Just beauty, inspired, pure, true

As you become more of the real you.